Praise for *Take Charge of Parkinson's Disease*

"Warmly and clearly written, *Take Charge of Parkinson's Disease* offers many healing, hopeful messages and invites readers to consider how meal times can become an essential part of the support system for persons with Parkinson's disease and their families. Nutritious, appealing, and comforting food is important for good mental health, emotional well-being, and better relationships in the face of chronic illness. The book applies evidence-based research to the role of nutrition, skillfully expressed through Anne's irresistible recipes and guidance for selecting 'brain healthy' ingredients. Through Anne's powerful storytelling and practical information about stress management, exercise, and caregiving, we are inspired to consider the things we can control: our outlook, what we eat, and the power of sharing our story with others. Simply reading this book is a healing experience for anyone touched by PD."

—Susan E. Ouellette, CRNP, CSP, APRN-PMH,
Psychiatric Nurse Practitioner and Patient Advocate

"The meaning of life is not where-you-get-to-in-the-end, but rather, the journey you take along the way. Anne Mikkelsen's book describes the bitter, sweet, complicated, funny, and very human path that she and her husband have followed for almost 30 years with Parkinson's disease. For any couple whose journey has screeched to a halt because of a diagnosis of Parkinson's disease, this book should be inspirational; it gives you permission—and some specific ideas about how—to regain control of your lives. And there are some great recipes for healthy foods included!"

—Martha A. Nance, MD, Medical Director,
Struthers Parkinson's Center, Minneapolis, MN

" ... an honest and inspiring story of one couple's journey with Parkinson's disease, filled with the power of hope and taking control of your life in a very practical way. The resilient attitude of Anne and Mike as they make changes to face day-to-day challenges provides a road map for others in similar situations.

The advice is very down to earth and doable, with clear suggestions about how to take charge of your diet, beginning with the introduction of 'the brain healthy pantry.' Numerous healthy, interesting, easy and mouthwatering recipes entice you to run to the kitchen and start cooking."

—Margaret Anne Coles, OTR/L, BSR, MQI,
Muhammad Ali Parkinson Center,
Barrow Neurological Institute, Phoenix, AZ

"*Take Charge of Parkinson's Disease* is an inspiring, must-read book for those caring for a loved one with the illness and for anyone interested in cognitive fitness and healthy aging. The authors clearly explain Parkinson's pathology—enabling caregivers to become more patient and supportive—then introducing readers to the 'brain-healthy pantry' and recipes that benefit brain health. Mikkelsen's simple, wholesome recipes are accessible to everyone; no special culinary skills are required, and her touching and sometimes humorous personal stories will surely add motivation and hope to the lives of millions challenged with the disease.

—Tina Ruggiero, M.S., R.D., L.D., Author of
The Best Homemade Baby Food on the Planet

"Concise, well-rounded, and up-to-date, with practical advice on living well with Parkinson's disease. I wish I'd had this book when I was diagnosed."

—Peter Dunlap-Shohl, Parkinson's Support Group Leader and Blogger,
Off and On: The Alaska Parkinson's Rag

"I couldn't put it down. This book makes people proactive and stresses early detection. The information is clear, short, to the point … and uplifting. And, the recipes are great! It's a book that especially people still 'in denial' should read."

—Barbe Awalt, whose father's struggle with Parkinson's disease
was chronicled in *The Stranger Comes At Sundown:
Living & Dying With Parkinson's Disease*

Take Charge of Parkinson's Disease

Dynamic Lifestyle Changes to Put *YOU* in the Driver's Seat

Take Charge of Parkinson's Disease

Dynamic Lifestyle Changes to Put *YOU* in the Driver's Seat

Anne Cutter Mikkelsen
with
Carolyn Stinson

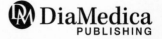 DiaMedica
PUBLISHING

DiaMedica Publishing, 150 East 61st Street, New York, NY 10065

Visit our website at www.diamedicapub.com

DiaMedica titles are available for bulk purchase, special promotions, and premiums. For more information please contact the publisher through the publisher's website: www.diamedicapub.com.

Disclaimer
The content in this book is not intended as a substitute for medical or professional counseling and advice. The reader is encouraged to consult his or her physicians and therapists on all health matters, especially symptoms that may require professional diagnosis and/or medical attention.

ISBN: 978-0-9823219-3-5

Cover design by Gopa & Ted2
Design by TypeWriting
Editing by Jessica Bryan, Joann Woy

Dedication

This book is dedicated to Mike Mikkelsen, for his courage and perseverance in making his voice heard, and to all people with Parkinson's disease. The energy behind your smiles could light the universe; your tender hearts and determination inspire compassion in those of us who look up to you every day.

May your muscles be peaceful, your brain relaxed and calm
May your doorways be spacious and your jokes be understood
May the weight lift from your shoulders when you lie down to sleep
May you live long and well with purpose
And someone by your side

And to our families:

Carolyn Stinson: To my husband Ken, for the space, advice, and encouragement to pursue and enjoy this adventure, several years in the making—and to my children, Jeffrey and Christine, for sharing their professional selves and enthusiasm in ways that enriched the material for this book.

Anne Mikkelsen: We hope the message in this book will add options to the lives of our children and positively affect the future for our grandchildren. Mike's: Jeremy, Vibeka, Annika, Maija, Amanda, and Sarah Elizabeth, and mine: Skye Olivia, Chelsea, Cutter, CharlaAnne, Ted, Aidan, Carmen, Isaac, Rohan, and Xereyna—and to the memory of Kenneth Larson, my children's grandfather, who lived with Parkinson's disease for 15 years.

*In memory of Tina Torrance, Bill Bell's mother
and inspiration for the Northwest Parkinson's Foundation.*

Acknowledgments

Committed to the message of our book, Carolyn Stinson led this project with insights and encouragement, sustaining our efforts from the start. Through Carolyn's diligence, our work captured the interest of a publisher.

We are grateful to our publisher, Diana M. Schneider, Ph.D., for her guidance, support, and energy, and for the opportunity to deliver the timely and compelling messages in this book.

Nanette J. Davis, Ph.D., sociologist and author, contributed a gem of a section: *When a Spouse Becomes a Caregiver*, which is a potent example of her understanding of caregiving.

Thank you Bill Bell for your poignant contribution to our project and your steadfast dedication to improving the quality of life for all people with Parkinson's disease.

We are grateful to Jay L. Alberts, Ph.D., Department of Biomedical Engineering and Center for Neurological Restoration at the Cleveland Clinic, for sharing his fascinating research on the effects of forced exercise and Parkinson's disease.

Thank you Geri Surratt for the exquisite botanical illustration of rosemary.

The most successful caregiving networks include family, friends, neighbors, and medical professionals. Mike was lucky to find Dr. Goo, a primary care doctor with old-fashioned values.

Our sincere gratitude goes to Anne's sisters, Acey, Milo, Liz, and Sarah, for their recipe testing and enthusiasm in helping us promote our message.

Contents

Part II: Food and Optimal Wellness with Parkinson's Disease

Foreword

There are two passions in my life. My first is Parkinson's disease. Or, more appropriately, it's helping those touched by Parkinson's to live their highest possible quality of life. For this, I can thank my mother, Tina Torrance. She was diagnosed with Parkinson's disease 26 years ago, at the young age of 46. Throughout her journey with Parkinson's, we have sought those strategies that allow her optimal quality of life—both with and without a doctor's prescription. We let the doctors take care of the clinical care, and we look for tools that will improve our self-care. This book in one of those tools.

My second passion is food—eating, making, trying, and discussing. When I travel, it's not from museum to historical site. It's restaurant to deli and back to restaurant. In retrospect, I can also most certainly thank my mother for this passion surrounding food. She has written two wonderful cookbooks, wrote restaurant reviews for various publications, ran a successful catering business, and has that innate ability to know what makes food taste good. Meals at home were not to be missed.

Take Charge of Parkinson's Disease blends both passions. It illustrates the benefits that we can bring to our lives through proper attitude, diet, and partnerships. So many times, we focus too much on the traditional clinical care rather than think about how we might feel better using available self-care tools. This book, with its insights and recipes, is a wonderful self-care tool that we can all benefit from. With an emphasis on wellness rather than diet, and healthy foods that can be presented with culinary art, this book will satisfy every appetite. Even my mother's.

William L. Bell
Former Executive Director
Northwest Parkinson's Foundation

Preface

M y husband Mike was born an artist of clay and steel, but when he was diagnosed with Parkinson's disease (PD) in 1993 our lives changed dramatically. I was trained as a chef in France at the dawn of the butter/cream foodie revolution. Together, we accepted the challenge to adapt our skills and adjust our lifestyle to include healthier food, more exercise, and maintain the creation of art. How did we get from pre-diagnosis to where we are now?

One of the primary purposes in writing this book is to spread the excitement and array of our newly discovered low-fat, brain-healthy pantry. In addition, I look forward to introducing you to some possibilities for delicious, savory meals loaded with antioxidants and anti-inflammatory substances known to benefit brain health. Through our story and compilation of 80-plus recipes, we hope to inspire you to stock your pantry well and create your own recipes using the dynamic list of colorful nutritional ingredients.

In our personal story, *Passion, Risk, Reward*, you'll learn about our bumpy, uninformed path through the initial stages of PD; how we built the perfect habitat: an energy-efficient home and a vibrant life in Northfield, Minnesota, and why we had to leave.

The food and magic of a small *casita* (cottage) by the sea in Kino Bay, Mexico, provided a perfect transition for Mike's healing to begin. His healing continued in Bellingham, Washington, where we designed our present home in anticipation of the future stages of PD.

Welcome to a virtual slideshow of Mike's outdoor sculptures and the symbolism associated with each work of art. We'll also take you inside the 2006

First World Parkinson's Congress in Washington D.C. There, you'll hear a doctor's sensitive observations about how our Parkinson's community works together toward the success of every member.

Woven throughout the narrative, you will find useful information regarding PD, contributed by Carolyn Stinson, including risk factors, symptoms, stages, and more. Carolyn's research is presented in a friendly and readable style, beginning with general information describing PD, and moving on to more nuanced signs and symptoms, including difficulty in diagnosis. What do we need to know about the causes of PD? What can you expect down the road if you've just been diagnosed? What is on the horizon for PD research?

Deftly blending the most current science with our journey through the stages of PD, Carolyn also discusses the common characteristics of depression, loss, stress, and anxiety.

Nanette J. Davis, Ph.D.—sociologist and author of *Blessed Is She: Women's Stories of Choice, Challenge and Commitment*—reflects on our story and gives us her perspective on successful caregiving in the section titled: "When a Spouse Becomes a Caregiver." What challenges do couples face, and how do they safely navigate the unfamiliar circumstances encountered in PD, with optimum results? Nanette outlines a simple strategy for "what works," focusing on the long-term rewards of caregiving rather than the burdens of care.

Exercise is essential to the success of the brain-healthy-lifestyle formula. What happens to the brain during exercise and why is exercise important for people with PD? Mike and I share what we've learned about our separate choices of exercise—including Mike's initial stubborn resistance and what changed his attitude.

The most empowering message we heard along the way was that, if we dared, we could take control of PD by changing our lifestyle. You will see how we ultimately learned to move Parkinson's to the back seat so we could see the road ahead.

Every day, at least three times a day, *we are in control.* The tools we need to protect our brains are right in our grocery store. What are those tools? What are free radicals, and how do antioxidants work in our bodies?

Throughout the stages of PD, Mike has gradually rewired his brain, and he is convinced that our lifestyle choices are responsible for the exceptional quality of life he enjoys today.

My hope is that readers will gain knowledge and understanding from our PD learning curve, save precious time, avoid unnecessary pitfalls, and add many quality-filled years to their lives.

Anne Cutter Mikkelsen

Introduction

WHAT IS PARKINSON'S DISEASE?*

Parkinson's disease (PD) is one of a group of medical conditions called *movement disorders*. It is the second most common progressive neurodegenerative disorder after Alzheimer's disease, and the second most prevalent and disabling condition in the expanding elderly population. At present, 1 percent of people over 50 have PD. Although the average age of onset is 60, increased awareness of the disease and advances in technology now allow neurologists to diagnose PD more easily in younger individuals. A diagnosis before age 40 is referred to as *young-onset Parkinson's disease* (YOPD).

PD is a chronic, progressive neurologic disorder that results from degeneration of neurons in a part of the brain called the *substantia nigra*, which controls muscle movement and coordination. This degeneration creates a shortage of the neurotransmitter *dopamine*, one of a group of substances responsible for communication between nerve cells. This, in turn, causes the impaired movement that characterizes the disease. Dopamine is responsible for transmitting signals between the substantia nigra and many other brain regions.

Other neurochemical changes in PD contribute to emotional and behavioral changes, sleep dysfunction, changes in cognitive function, and pain. As

---

* This chapter presents general information about Parkinson's disease. It is not intended as a scientific, technical, or comprehensive treatment of the subject matter. The Resources section includes references to more technical material; we especially recommend *Parkinson's Disease: A Complete Guide for Patients and Families*.

these dopamine-producing cells begin to die, the amount of dopamine produced in the brain decreases. Scientists believe that by the time clinical symptoms are apparent, a significant proportion of the cells in the substantia nigra, 60–80 percent, may already have been destroyed.

The symptoms and disease progression in PD vary widely among individuals and, over time, often cause considerable disability and reduction in quality of life. Parkinson's disease can produce a wide variety of unpredictable symptoms that affect many systems of the body. Its cause remains unknown, and there is no known cure. However, significant advances have been made in therapies that offer relief from symptoms.

A HISTORY OF PARKINSON'S DISEASE

Parkinson's disease is named after the English apothecary James Parkinson, who provided a detailed description of the disease in his 1817 publication, *An Essay on the Shaking Palsy.*

The disorder has been recognized since ancient times. For example, it is referred to as *Kampavata*, for "tremor," in the ancient Indian medical system of Ayurveda. In Western medical literature, the physician Galen described it as "shaking palsy" in 175 A.D.

Despite the longstanding awareness of PD, the chemical differences in the brains of people with PD were identified only as recently as the 1960s, with the discovery of low dopamine levels and the link to the degeneration of nerve cells in the substantia nigra. This discovery led to the first effective treatment of the disease—the drug *levodopa*, which has since become the "gold standard" in medication.

WHO IS AFFECTED BY PARKINSON'S DISEASE?

More than one million people in the United States are living with PD, more than the number of people diagnosed with multiple sclerosis, muscular dystrophy, and Lou Gehrig's disease combined. Approximately 60,000–70,000 people are diagnosed with PD each year in the United States.

Men have a 1.5 times greater risk than do women for developing PD. Epidemiologic studies suggest that its incidence can vary by race, ethnicity, and geography, even within the United States. Six million people are affected among the 15 largest nations worldwide, and this number is projected to grow to 8.7 million by the year 2030.

Young-Onset Parkinson's Disease

Young-onset Parkinson's disease accounts for 5–10 percent of the total number of people with PD. Although some evidence suggests that people with YOPD have a slower disease progression and lower incidence of dementia, they have psychosocial issues that require as much attention as medical ones. In many respects, they must deal with greater challenges than do older individuals. They are diagnosed during the most productive years of their lives, face decades of life with the illness, and may have dependent children or are caring for older family members.

WHAT CAUSES PARKINSON'S DISEASE?

Parkinson's disease is referred to as an *idiopathic* disease, which means that it has no known cause, but there are probably a number of causal factors involved in its development. Although researchers cannot pinpoint a single cause of PD, several primary risk factors have been identified. These include advancing age, genetic susceptibility, and environmental factors that lead to neurodegeneration and cell loss. Several so-called "mechanisms of cell death" are suspect in the accelerated aging and death of the neurons that produce dopamine. Evidence for several of these "cell death pathways" has been found in the brains of PD patients.

Many scientists think the primary reason why neurons die in PD is chronic *inflammation*, which has been referred to as "the engine that drives the

Parkinson's disease process." Inflammation is part of a process by which the body's immune system protects against infection and foreign substances such as viruses and bacteria. Although inflammation is part of the body's normal response to such harmful agents, and it is essential for survival, too much can be harmful.

People with PD also progressively lose the nerve endings that produce the neurotransmitter *norepinephrine*, the main chemical messenger of the *sympathetic nervous system*. This part of the nervous system—the *autonomic* nervous system—regulates unconscious, or involuntary, bodily functions, including heart rate, blood pressure, temperature, gastrointestinal processes, and metabolic and endocrine responses. The loss of norepinephrine, therefore, might help explain several of the features of PD that are not related to movement, such as fatigue and a slowing of the rate at which food moves through the digestive tract.

Age

Age is the greatest risk factor for the development and progression of PD, probably because it affects many of the cellular processes that can lead to neurodegeneration. These are believed by researchers to include increased oxidative stress, mitochondrial damage, and vulnerability to inflammation, all of which seem to be part of the normal aging process.

Genetics

Only a very small percentage of PD cases have been identified as genetically related, meaning that the disease is present in a disproportionately high number of family members; these cases are considered *familial Parkinson's disease*. Several different gene mutations have been definitively linked to PD, including a few that cause the rare young-onset form of PD. In early 2010, a new genetic risk factor for PD was identified that points to the interaction of genetic and environmental factors such as dietary habits.

Environmental Factors

Some epidemiologic evidence suggests that environmental toxins may play a role in the development of PD, but as yet none has been confirmed. These might include pesticides, solvents, metals such as lead and mercury, contaminants in food, and exposure to infectious agents. The incidence of PD varies geographically, which provides some support for these findings. For example, rural areas with farming and widespread consumption of well water have been associated with an increased risk of developing PD. Occupational exposure to certain groups of herbicides, pesticides, and insecticides also may to be associated with as much as a 70 percent increased chance of developing PD, according to some researchers.

Secondary Parkinson's or "Parkinsonism"

The term *secondary Parkinson's disease*, or *secondary parkinsonism*, refers to individuals who show certain symptoms of PD, but the symptoms are caused by a different problem, such as head trauma, brain tumor, stroke, or another nervous system disorder. For example, *postencephalitic parkinsonism* is caused by a virus, and can lead to a severe form of movement disorder years after the initial illness. Secondary parkinsonism can also be caused by medication side effects that are not connected with the drugs or therapies used to treat PD.

Several studies have indicated that head trauma substantially increases the risk of PD. Laboratory studies have demonstrated that chronic head injury impairs energy metabolism and increases oxidative stress and neuroinflammation. Understandably, there is a correlation between head trauma and chronic head injury, as in boxing, with an increased risk of developing PD.

Depression As a Possible Risk Factor for Parkinson's Disease

Depression may have important implications in PD, both as a risk factor and as a consequence of the disease. Some researchers believe that depression is actually part of the core condition of PD. People with PD are at a higher than average risk for developing depression. It occurs in about 40 percent of individuals at some point during the illness, double the incidence seen in the general population.

Depression is common in most chronic neurologic disorders, however, affecting 20–50 percent of people with stroke, multiple sclerosis, epilepsy, dementia, Alzheimer's disease, and PD. However, despite these significant numbers, the cause of depression in neurologic disorders is not straightforward. It has been attributed to several factors, including the person's emotional reaction to dealing with the diagnosis and disability, the neurochemical impact of neurodegeneration, and the influence of other disease factors.

Diagnosing depression in the context of a neurologic disorder is challenging, and the symptoms of depression can overlap those of the neurologic disorder.

Depression in PD has even further-reaching effects, because it can increase the likelihood of depression in caregivers. It can also increase the incidence of other chronic illnesses.

Mood disorders might also be a cause of neurodegeneration. Researchers have reported an association between depression and anxiety disorders, and the eventual onset of PD. A history of depression of up to 10 years duration appears to be significantly associated with the development of PD. Even an "anxious personality" that started many years before the onset of clinical symptoms may be associated with development of PD. Chronic psychological stress has also been shown to trigger adverse physiologic changes that contribute to cell death. The details of a possible association between mood disorders and the eventual development of PD are as yet unknown. It is also possible that this apparent association is a side issue and there is no causal relationship.

SIGNS AND SYMPTOMS OF PARKINSON'S DISEASE

Parkinson's disease produces a constellation of symptoms that are categorized as either *motor* or *non-motor*. The term *motor* symptom refers to the effects of

PD on movement. These are the symptoms that most people commonly associate with PD.

Motor Symptoms

The first early indication of PD is often a *resting* tremor, which appears when a limb is at rest and disappears when it is moved. However, 30 percent of people with PD do not have tremor at the onset of the disease; others develop tremor at some point during the progression of their illness—or not at all. Several other types of tremors may also occur.

The first motor symptoms typically appear on only one side of the body, and it can be years before the other side is affected. Even when both sides are involved, symptoms usually remain more pronounced on the side that was first affected. The early symptoms can be so subtle and occur so gradually that they are often not noticed or are dismissed. Even after diagnosis, the disease can progress slowly for several years before symptoms intensify to the point of causing serious dysfunction and disability.

People with PD may experience a wide variation in the types and severity of symptoms. One person might experience only a few symptoms, even for a period of years—others may need to deal with multiple symptoms at the same time. The time spent in each stage of the disease varies, and skipping stages is not uncommon. The *Hoehn and Yahr Scale* is a rating system used by physicians to follow the severity of a person's symptoms and progression of the disease. It is divided into five stages:

> **Stage 1:** Symptoms are mild and may be present on just one side of the body; daily tasks of living may be somewhat more difficult to perform; there may be tremor in one limb or on one side of the body; and some physical changes may be apparent to others, including poor posture, problems with balance, unusual facial expressions, or problems with speech.

Common *motor* or movement-related symptoms of Parkinson's disease (PD) include:

▶ Tremor, or shaking, often in a hand, arm, or leg. Tremor caused by PD occurs when the person is awake and sitting or standing still (resting tremor) and subsides when the person intentionally moves the affected body part. Sleep or complete relaxation usually stops or reduces the tremor. One-third of people with PD do not experience tremor.

▶ Slow, limited movement (*bradykinesia*), especially when the person tries to move from a resting position. For instance, it may be difficult to get out of a chair or turn over in bed.

▶ Stiff muscles (*rigidity*) and aching muscles. One of the most common early signs of PD is reduced arm swing on one side when the person is walking, caused by rigid muscles. Rigidity can also affect the muscles of the legs, face, neck, or other parts of the body.

▶ Difficulty with walking (*gait disturbance*) and balance (*postural instability*); a sudden inability to move, usually involving walking, which can last for seconds or much longer (*freezing*). A person with PD is likely to take shuffling, small steps and bend forward slightly at the waist.

▶ Weakness of face and throat muscles. Talking and swallowing may become more difficult, and the person may choke, cough, or drool. There may be trouble swallowing and excessive salivation. Speech becomes softer and monotonous. Loss of movement in the muscles in the face can cause a fixed, vacant facial expression, often called the *Parkinson's mask*, *masked face*, or *facial mask*. An inability to smile or blink may also be present.

▶ Decreased dexterity and coordination. Athletic abilities decline, and daily activities such as dressing and eating become more difficult.

▶ Painful, twisting muscle contractions, frequently in the foot and ankle, a condition called *dystonia*.

▶ Small, cramped handwriting, or *micrographia*.

▶ Restlessness or an inability to sit or lie still, referred to as *akathisia*.

Having at least two of these symptoms strongly suggests a diagnosis of PD.

Stage 2: Tremor and other motor symptoms affect both sides of the body; problems walking or maintaining balance have developed; and normal daily physical tasks have become increasingly difficult.

Stage 3: Symptoms become severe and can include the inability to walk straight or stand; a stooped posture is common; and physical movements are noticeably stiff and much slower.

Stage 4: The ability to walk is often limited, and rigidity and bradykinesia are often apparent. Most people in Stage 4 are unable to handle activities of daily living (ADLs); they require assistance or may not be able to live alone. Although the reason is not understood, tremors may lessen temporarily during this stage.

Stage 5: People who have reached this stage are usually unable to care for themselves and may not be able to stand or walk; they usually require one-on-one care; and speech may be severely affected.

Parkinson's disease symptoms are difficult to predict and control. From day to day—even hour-to-hour—a person may experience wide fluctuations in the severity and type of symptoms. This can be caused by factors other than the disease itself, such as medications and psychological stress. Managing unpredictable symptoms can be frustrating. People must continually adapt their daily routine in order to accommodate changing symptoms, as well as make frequent adjustments to the dosage and timing of their medications.

Parkinson's disease presents daily challenges and stressors for everyone concerned—the person with PD, caregivers, and other family members. Parkinson's disease symptoms that can be observed by others are often troubling and embarrassing, leading to social withdrawal, depression, and relationship problems. Stress and anxiety can vary with fluctuations in motor performance and, conversely, most people notice an increase in motor symptoms during periods of high anxiety.

Non-Motor Symptoms

Parkinson's disease is not *just* a movement disorder. A high percentage of people with PD—nearly 90 percent—experience non-motor disturbances that can be a significant source of distress, disability, and decreased quality of life. These include sensory, autonomic, cognitive, emotional/behavioral, and sleep-related changes.

Non-motor symptoms can result from the disease process itself, but they can also be a consequence of the medications needed to manage PD.

Until recently, non-motor symptoms were often under-recognized, under-appreciated, and under-treated, despite their significant impact on quality of life. Increasingly, education and growing self-awareness are helping people

---

Non-motor symptoms (those unrelated to movement) can include:

▶ Pain and various forms and degrees of physical discomfort

▶ Emotional and mood changes, including depression, apathy, anxiety, and problems with impulse control, including obsessive-compulsive behaviors

▶ Difficulty concentrating; diminished mental energy; memory loss; confusion

▶ Fatigue

▶ Cramps in muscles and joints

▶ Oily skin; increased dandruff; rashes

▶ Reduction in or loss of sense of smell

▶ Constipation; difficulty controlling urination

▶ Poor digestion

▶ Problems with involuntary or automatic body functions, such as increased sweating, low blood pressure when the person stands up, and sexual function

▶ Insomnia or problems falling asleep

▶ Dementia

with PD, physicians, and caregivers to link certain signs and symptoms with the disease. This has prompted exploration of new therapies and interventions. Some non-motor symptoms cause more pervasive and troublesome problems than others. Particular emphasis has been placed on the treatment of pain, a frequent but still under-reported symptom.

Recognizing non-motor changes as soon as possible, however subtle they may be, is important because they can precede the onset of motor symptoms. For example, a reduction or loss of the sense of smell is a frequent symptom that some research indicates may be a very early feature of PD, foreshadowing the appearance of motor symptoms by years.

Pain

Pain is reported by at least 50 percent of people with PD, and it is significantly more common compared to the general population. For some people, pain can be more debilitating than movement dysfunction.

Pain syndromes and discomfort can result from a number of causes, including:

- ▶ A musculoskeletal problem—aching muscles and joints—related to poor posture, awkward mechanical function, or physical wear and tear
- ▶ Nerve or nerve root pain, often related to arthritis in the neck or back
- ▶ Pain from dystonia, which involves sustained twisting or posturing of a muscle group or body part
- ▶ Extreme restlessness
- ▶ A rare pain syndrome known as "primary" or "central" pain that originates from within the nervous system

Pain can also be associated with either inadequate or high levels of dopamine receptor stimulation, in which case management includes adjusting anti-parkinsonian medication.

Sleep

Sleep is essential to everyone's good health and sense of well-being. However, sleep quality is a major source of dissatisfaction for two-thirds or more of people with PD. Sleep is often light and fragmented, and difficulty maintaining sleep throughout the night is one of the most commonly reported problems. Other sleep disturbances include insomnia, early morning awakening, vivid dreams and nightmares, and frequent nighttime urination. Disrupted sleep contributes to the excessive daytime sleepiness experienced by many people with PD. A number of causes are implicated in sleep dysfunction in PD, including psychological stress, depression and anxiety, *sleep apnea*, involuntary movements, pain, difficulty turning or changing position, and uncomfortable sensations in the legs. Drugs used to treat PD can also contribute to sleep problems.

DIAGNOSING PARKINSON'S DISEASE

Diagnosing PD is not always straightforward, especially in the early stages, when symptoms may not be obvious. A high rate of misdiagnosis also occurs. This is true for a number of reasons, including:

- ▶ There is no laboratory or blood test to diagnose PD, and no single factor or symptom has been determined as a diagnostic marker. Diagnosis is based on an individual's medical history, a thorough physical examination, clinical observation over time, and the ruling out of other medical disorders using diagnostic imaging, brain scans, and other tests.
- ▶ Denial is a common reaction when a person first experiences symptoms that could be associated with PD, and they do not always report their symptoms to their family or health care provider.
- ▶ Early signs and symptoms may go unnoticed or be dismissed as the effects of normal aging.

▶ A diagnosis of PD is assumed if a person has at least two of the principal motor symptoms of PD. One-sided, or predominantly one-sided, symptoms also are important clues.

▶ Often, a person suspected of having PD will be given the drug *levodopa*; if symptoms improve or disappear, the diagnosis is confirmed.

The Unified Parkinson's Disease Rating Scale (UPDRS) is a comprehensive symptom questionnaire used by neurologists or movement disorders specialists during the medical examination and history phase of diagnosis. Neurologists and researchers also use this tool in clinical practice to follow disease progression, study symptoms, and measure benefit from therapies. The UPDRS encompasses the Hoehn and Yahr Scale, described above.

TREATMENT AND SYMPTOM MANAGEMENT

Parkinson's disease treatment is largely symptomatic because there is no known cure. Medications can lose their effectiveness over a period of years. For this reason, drug treatment may not be appropriate in the early stages of the disease if symptoms are mild and do not interfere too much with daily activities. It is often preferable to delay drug therapy until symptoms begin to cause more serious issues.

At any stage of the disease, exercise and physical, speech, and occupational therapy can be helpful in maintaining strength, mobility, and independence. Physical therapy can help improve range of motion and muscle tone. Emerging evidence suggests that certain types of regular exercise may delay the appearance of some symptoms, and even slow, stop, or reverse neurodegeneration, and possibly promote neurorestoration. Exercise also has a beneficial impact on depression, sleep quality, and cognitive function.

Other non-pharmacologic strategies can alleviate symptoms and empower patients and their families, including:

▶ Stress management
▶ Treating depression and anxiety
▶ Developing coping skills
▶ Improving sleep hygiene
▶ Good nutrition
▶ Cultivating a support network

A strong relationship exists between social support and psychological health in people with PD—those with inadequate social support often have a higher incidence of depression, anxiety, and stress.

Medications

Pharmacologic therapy for PD involves medications that balance dopamine levels in the nervous system, including levodopa, carbidopa, and dopamine agonists.

Levodopa, also called *L-Dopa*, has been the main drug therapy for PD for many decades. This substance is naturally present in the body. Nerve cells use levodopa to make dopamine, which replenishes the dopamine lost because of neurodegeneration and cell loss.

Levodopa is usually taken in combination with *carbidopa*, which assists in the process of converting levodopa into dopamine. Carbidopa protects levodopa from prematurely converting to dopamine outside of the brain, which prevents or reduces some of the side effects of levodopa therapy, which might include nausea, confusion, delusions and hallucinations, rapid heart rate, and involuntary writhing movements called *dyskinesias*. Dyskinesias occur more commonly after an extended period of treatment with levodopa, and may involve the arms, legs, hands, face, mouth, or neck. They can also mean that too much medication is being used, in which case adjustments to dosage and timing may be indicated. Another advantage of using carbidopa in combination with levodopa is that the total daily dose of levodopa may be lowered.

Many experts recommend *dopamine agonists* as an alternative to levodopa-carbidopa therapy. Dopamine agonists activate dopamine receptors and mimic, or copy, the function of dopamine in the brain. They are often better tolerated and do not have the same risk of long-term complications as levodopa therapy. For these reasons, dopamine agonists are often the first choice of treatment for PD, particularly in younger, healthier individuals. If a person's symptoms cannot be controlled sufficiently with a dopamine agonist, levodopa can be added.

Unfortunately, dopamine agonists may cause short-term side effects such as nausea, vomiting, dizziness, light-headedness, confusion, and hallucinations. They may also increase the risk of compulsive behaviors such as gambling, overeating, or hypersexuality.

Over time, medications often lose their effectiveness in controlling PD symptoms. Loss of efficacy of treatment with drugs and disturbing side effects are particularly challenging for people with young-onset PD, because they face many more years of managing symptoms. People who are diagnosed and begin treatment at an older age often find that medications can sustain their quality of life throughout their lifetime, by controlling symptoms without causing problems or complications.

When drug efficacy wanes or becomes inconsistent, or when side effects become intolerable, a neurosurgical intervention called *deep brain stimulation* (DBS) may be considered. Deep brain stimulation involves implanting a brain stimulator, similar to a heart pacemaker, in certain areas of the brain. Such a device can stabilize medication fluctuations and greatly reduce or eliminate dyskinesias. Tremor is especially responsive to this therapy. For some people, DBS may control symptoms so well that medications can be greatly reduced.

As with any surgical procedure, risks are associated with DBS; however, it is relatively safe. Deep brain stimulation blocks electrical impulses in targeted areas of the brain, but it does not purposefully destroy any part of the brain. The electrical stimulation it provides can be adjusted as needed—without additional surgery—as the disease progresses, or in response to changes in medications.

THE FUTURE

Researchers continue to look for predictive and diagnostic tools for PD, and for effective, noninvasive ways to prevent or slow progression of the disease.

Emerging scientific evidence suggests that certain types of exercise may be neuroprotective and offer symptom relief in PD. Research is also focused on nutrition for possible neuroprotection, including exploration of the antioxidant and anti-inflammatory potential in certain foods, dietary supplements, vitamins, and culinary spices and herbs. Managing the symptoms and progression of PD with these complementary strategies is the major focus of this book.

PART I

Passion, Risk, and Reward: Our Story

The Artist and the Chef

*Use your personal strengths to adapt to the changes
inherent in living with Parkinson's disease, and develop
coping strategies that work for you.*

Before Parkinson's disease (PD), Mike and I were "the Artist and the Chef."
We are still the Artist and the Chef, but we have adapted our skills to current conditions and emerging science.

Living with PD is simultaneously gratifying and frustrating, rewarding and challenging. Through the lens of almost three decades of living with the disease, it's easy to track our learning curve. From this perspective, we recognize what almost destroyed our partnership, and what we are currently doing that contributes to our marital happiness and longevity.

I don't deny the difficulties, the dark months and years, as we fearfully fumbled through the first stages of Mike's PD. But fear cripples the brain, and dwelling on the negatives threatened to destroy all our positive intentions. Instead, we intuitively developed coping mechanisms that we hope will be useful to other people with PD and those who love and care for them. Over the years, our constants have included exercise, taking risks, maintaining our individual pursuits, and eating good food every day.

Mike had always been a pretty healthy guy, with the exception of a serious motorcycle accident in his 30s, when he suffered a concussion and had one leg completely severed. He didn't drink coffee until his 40s, and he's never been a smoker. He did take chances with his health, such as not protecting himself in his pottery studio while mixing glazes and clay formulas. For years, he welded and painted cars with no ventilation or protective gear.

The diagnosis that Mike had suspected for 12 years was confirmed in 1993, at the Mayo Clinic. When he asked for a prognosis, I almost covered my ears. The doctor responded cautiously, "Of course every case is different," he explained, "but you will probably need *serious* care in 10 years." To us, *serious care* was code for a wheelchair and diapers. Seventeen years after that prediction, Mike is 77. He still walks a mile every morning, participates in yoga classes twice a week, reads every night, eats everything he enjoys, drives his '41 Dodge convertible whenever he desires, and—most importantly—Mike is still creating his art.

Along the way, we learned—through trial and error—about the importance of healthy coping strategies and the critical need for regular exercise and good nutrition.

Healthy Coping Strategies

Healthy coping skills help people adapt, manage stress, and boost their physical and emotional resilience. Not all coping behaviors are healthy, however, such as withdrawing from family and friends. It takes serious effort to avoid behaviors that can have a negative impact on your life. Here are some positive coping strategies.

▶ Recognizing that you have power over how you think about Parkinson's disease (PD) and its effect on your life. Avoid thinking in extremes such as, "my life is over," or "my life will not change because of PD."

▶ Protecting your relationship with your spouse or significant other. Consider couples counseling early in the course of the disease, and choose a therapist who has experience in supporting couples dealing with the challenges of a chronic disease.

▶ Beginning interventions early to
  • Recognize and treat depression and anxiety in both you and your partner
  • Maintain optimal nutrition
  • Include exercise and physical therapy
  • Practice memory training
  • Cope with speech, voice, and language changes

▶ Staying in touch with family and friends, and maintaining an active social life. Withdrawal and isolation are major psychological stressors for people with PD and their caregivers.

▶ Building a wide support network that includes your medical care team, financial and legal advisors, work colleagues, clergy, and support groups.

▶ Not abandoning hobbies or other pleasurable activities, and finding ways to work around limitations created by symptoms.

▶ Learning simple relaxation and meditation techniques, and putting them into practice on a daily basis.

▶ Finding ways to nourish your spirit.

▶ Being open with your physician about symptoms and concerns.

▶ Establishing good sleep hygiene habits; for example, limiting daytime naps.

▶ Educating yourself about PD—information is empowering.

Exercise and Parkinson's Disease

Most people in the early stages of Parkinson's disease (PD) don't consider how exercise might be beneficial, possibly because they have not yet realized that their function has declined, or that the effects of the disease are beginning to interfere with the activities of daily life. Regular exercise is one of the most positive steps you can take to help manage the symptoms and progression of PD. It has certainly helped Mike and me.

Many health care providers fail to address the issue of exercise until 5 or more years after diagnosis, when more serious issues begin to arise. This misses a window of opportunity during which you can optimize your health so you will be better able to cope with symptoms.

Exercise can improve both the physical and mental issues that most people encounter with PD. Physically, it improves balance, muscle strength, posture, flexibility, and mobility. It also prevents joint stiffening. Emotionally, exercise has beneficial effects on stress, mood, depression and anxiety, cognitive decline, and sleep quality.

Some of the key observations that have been made about the benefits of exercise in PD are:

▶ Regular exercise appears to delay the appearance of *parkinsonian* features in people who have already been diagnosed.
▶ Inactivity may contribute to loss of function and disease progression.
▶ Certain types of frequent, intense exercise—fast moving with high repetition, for example—can alter the way the brain works and may slow, stop, or even reverse the progression of PD by promoting neuroprotection.

Low-impact exercise such as tai chi, qigong (chi-gong), yoga, and treadmill training are recommended for people with PD to help improve impaired coordination and balance.

- ▶ Tai chi was developed in China more than 1,000 years ago, and uses slow, graceful movement to relax and strengthen muscles and joints. This form of exercise provides benefits for people in all stages of PD, including improvements in cardiovascular fitness.
- ▶ Qigong incorporates meditation, movement, and sometimes breathing techniques.
- ▶ Yoga uses gentle stretching and meditation to relax tense muscles and relieve mental stress.
- ▶ Treadmill training has emerged recently as a promising investigational therapy that may improve gait speed, stride length, and walking distance.

Leaving Minnesota

Denial of early symptoms can cause unnecessary anxiety.
There is no need to suffer in silence.

Even though he wasn't diagnosed with Parkinson's disease (PD) until 1993, Mike suspected trouble much earlier. He believes his first symptoms emerged in 1981, the year after we were married, and the same year that we finished building our earth berm, passive-solar home on 40 acres in Northfield, Minnesota. Mike was the architect and general contractor. Our method of building the foundation was innovative and practically experimental at the time, but Mike convinced an engineer to sign-off on the plans and we moved forward with confidence.

Earth berm describes a style of building, usually constructed of concrete and built into a hillside, designed to take advantage of geothermal heat with the roof and one side exposed. Such homes are energy-efficient, low maintenance, and built to last over 100 years.

Three walls of our home were constructed with floor-to-ceiling dry-stacked concrete blocks, reinforced with steel bars and bonded with a newly developed cementitious (cement-like) material. Dirt was back-filled and terraced against the three walls from the ground to the edge of the roof. The exposed south-facing wall was a bank of windows designed for passive solar heating. The roof was exposed and built over four separate bays; the ceiling of each bay had two clerestories (small window-dormers) that captured the eastern light. To frame the roof, we used scissor trusses (roof superstructure) over each of the four bays to create high-vaulted or cathedral ceilings in each bay.

My four young children—Sean, 13; Geoffrey, 12; Andy, 10; and Sarah, 9—helped with every stage of building the house. Mike's lifelong buddy Skip helped us stack the concrete blocks, pour the concrete floors, frame the rooms, wire, plumb, and insulate our one-story, 3,400 square-foot "smart" house.

One especially invigorating early fall morning during construction, Mike and Skip created a table out of building materials in the spot that would eventually be Sarah's bedroom. The week before, the children had assisted us in setting the 48 scissor trusses for the roof, and today was their first day of school in Northfield. At this point, our new home had no interior walls—only three outside walls, a concrete floor, and the vaulted trusses open to the sky.

I unfolded my grandmother's linen and lace tablecloth over the plywood table-top. With a bouquet of wild flowers in the center, the three of us sat on cinder block chairs for a celebratory coffee break with warm poppy seed muffins and fresh fruit.

Poppy Seed Muffins
(Makes 6 muffins)

¼ pound unsalted butter
½ cup sugar
1 egg
¾ cup flour

¼ cup milk
1 T poppy seeds
½ tsp nutmeg, freshly grated

Topping

3 T unsalted butter, melted

4 T sugar mixed with 1 tsp cinnamon

Preheat oven to 350 degrees. Soften the butter and mix with sugar at high speed. When sugar and butter are well blended, add egg and beat until incorporated. Add half the flour and mix at medium speed. Add poppy seeds, milk, and nutmeg. Add remaining flour and mix until smooth.

Line muffin tin with papers and divide batter. Bake 25 minutes. Let cool a few minutes before removing muffins from papers.

Dip muffin tops into melted butter and then into sugar/cinnamon mixture. Serve with a plate of fresh fruit.

───────────

Shortly after completing our home, Mike, then 47-years old, was on the roof of a funky round house he was helping construct for an artist friend named Furry Foot. He couldn't figure out why his familiar, dependable speed square suddenly made no sense to him. No matter which way he placed the tool, it wasn't right. Maybe, he rationalized, it was the unusual design of Foot's house, not his own sudden inability to maneuver or understand the speed square.

Whatever the problem was, Mike did not tell me about this early warning until years later. During that time, he regularly and secretly consulted *The Mayo Clinic Patient Handbook*, tracking his mounting symptoms—stooped posture, difficulty walking, depression, and rigidity. For Mike, the most defining and irrefutable evidence that something was going on with his health was his diminutive handwriting, which had been reduced almost to a flat line by the time he was diagnosed. This is known as *micrographia*, and it's one of the most common symptoms of PD.

Stress and Parkinson's Disease

Stress can be alleviated with support from other people, so reach out to family and friends, and seek professional help, if necessary. Open communication is critical. Exercise and other complementary therapies can also help relieve stress.

People with Parkinson's disease (PD) have a lower tolerance for stress, and stress can severely impact their quality of life. People with PD frequently experience distress when others can observe their symptoms. As symptoms increase, they may experience a growing sense of alienation, which can lead to social isolation. In addition, most people with PD suffer sleep from disturbances. These two issues—social isolation and sleep disturbances—are major *psychological stressors*.

Individuals with young-onset PD often face stressors that are not typically shared by people who are diagnosed later in life. Loss of employment because of disability or early retirement, disruption of family life with young children, and more severe treatment-related motor complications can contribute to a greater perceived stigma associated with the disease.

Stress levels can be reduced by social interaction and support from family, friends, colleagues, and the community, and with the development of coping skills and exercise. Meditation, aromatherapy, massage, and traditional counseling or psychotherapy can be effective in managing stress.

Chronic psychological stress has many consequences. It can interfere with the effectiveness of PD medications, and can lead to anxiety
and depression. It is also linked to increased severity and intensity of
certain PD symptoms. Stress can also lead to greater distress in caregivers. Animal studies suggest that stress can even negate the neuroprotective benefits of nutrition and exercise.

Each individual experiences the symptoms of PD in different combinations, at
different times, and with varying degrees of intensity, frequency, and duration.
Lack of recognition or denial of symptoms can cause relationship and other
stress-related difficulties.

Mike did not share his discoveries with me for a long time, so I drew my
own conclusions from his obvious symptoms. He has never shown any tremor,
which in the early stages might have narrowed my considerations. Instead, for
years I feared depression or—worse—a brain tumor, but he preferred not to
discuss or consider treatment. Knowing Mike as well as I do now, I suspect he
knew where his health was headed.

The most divisive symptom was Mike's startling facial mask. He would
appear in the kitchen with an expression that seemed to say: "I'm miserable
and confused because of *you*, something *you've* done or neglected to do." His
lack of affect and our combined lack of knowledge about the source of his
stone-faced glares "stirred the pot to a boil" way too many times.

I now have a more educated view of the stress that PD created in our lives
and—with the perspective of time—I realize that abandoning a person who is
sinking into illness is *not* an option. Release from the quicksand requires more,
rather than fewer, helping hands. I also know that, on this side of PD, life has
become sweeter and filled with more tenderness because we made it through
the grittiness of "the rough sandpaper stages" and into the smooth finish.

Sweeter and more tender because we have reached a point at which Mike
needs me to help him communicate; some might view this as a burden, but
actually the ability to interpret Mike's needs through reading his body lan-

guage and observing his mounting anxiety is an intimate and loving exchange—an unexpected communion that has brought us closer than we have ever been. It is the best I have to offer. Even though he does not speak as much as he used to, he's still communicating. More and more often, Mike displays subtle signals for me to decode—a confused frown, a sentence uncompleted, agitated legs and feet, or overt signs like simply handing the phone to me with the hope that I will continue his conversation.

Our Northfield home was the bustling scene of hundreds of events centered on friends, family, art, and food. Mike built his new pottery studio and gas kiln across the yard, where he hosted sales twice a year. For these events, I prepared classic French pastries—crepes, brioche, and beignets with fillings and butter creams gilded with sauces made from fruit growing wild along our long drive-

During the 2006 elections, we watched Michael J. Fox on television endorsing Claire McCaskill for U.S. Senate. McCaskill, a Missouri Democrat, was an outspoken advocate for stem cell research. During the taping, Fox was besieged with dyskinesia (involuntary movement), a common side effect of Parkinson's medication, but he continued speaking.

As I watched him struggle through his message, I was proud of his class and courage. Michael J. Fox is a leader in the PD community. He has put his private life and vulnerability on public display in the best interests of millions of people with Parkinson's all over the world.

It's easy to see why people with PD, especially those with young-onset PD, might perceive a stigma associated with their disease. If they have the courage to take a chance, avoid isolation, and appear in public under unpredictable circumstances, they might be judged by their appearance, their uncontrollable movements, or their lack of movement. Their motives might be questioned and ridiculed by people with little or no education about PD—and so their stress levels rise, dopamine levels plummet, and the downward cycle continues.

way—plums, gooseberries, and raspberries. We served these sweet morsels on Mike's porcelain platters, with sauces poured from his stoneware pitchers.

Here is a good example of the treats we served our pottery customers.

Strawberries Nougatine

For the Caramel Nougatine

½ cup slivered almonds   3 T water

⅓ cup sugar

For the Strawberries

8–10 strawberries per person   1 cup whipped cream

1 T sugar   1 T sugar

2 tsp orange zest   2 tsp vanilla

1 T Grand Marnier liqueur

To create the nougatine, warm almonds in the oven at 350 degrees for about 7 minutes. Lightly oil a baking sheet. Combine sugar and water in small enameled saucepan or copper caramel pan. Bring caramel to a boil. When it reaches a light brown color, add warmed almonds. Stir and quickly pour onto oiled baking sheet. Let cool. When cooled, transfer nougatine to a food processor and chop to small chunks.

Clean 8–10 strawberries per person. In a large bowl, sprinkle strawberries with a little sugar and orange zest. Drizzle with Grand Marnier and let stand for an hour. Whip some cream with sugar and vanilla.

Arrange strawberries on individual plates. Top with whipped cream and sprinkle with nougatine.

Restoring vintage automobiles has been one of Mike's artistic endeavors since acquiring his first Model T at the age of 8 on his parents' ranch in Montana. "Rolling sculptures," he reverently calls them. In his lifetime, he's owned more than 200 "cars of interest."

In his Northfield pottery studio, Mike built a trap door with a ladder down to the garage, with an ample paint booth below. He frequently slipped away from his pottery wheel and went down that ladder, spending hours pounding and shaping metal, welding, assembling, painting, and restoring over 50 vintage cars.

With acres of bare land around us, I decided to uncover the secrets of how "real people" built and maintained beautiful gardens—without having to pull weeds. I completed Master Gardener training only to discover that real people pull weeds! We planted hundreds of trees and constructed flowerbeds from cherished gifts bestowed by friends and neighbors. We surrounded our gardens with walls of native limestone, hauled up stone by stone from an old chicken coop at the bottom of our hill.

Nothing was more satisfying than creating our garden borders from indigenous found material. We worked in the spring rain until almost dark, with the comforting scent of a savory chicken roasting in the kitchen to keep us company. With the kitchen window slightly open, we worked harder and faster, anticipating the meal that would be waiting.

Oven-roasted Chicken with Indian Spices and Lemons

One 3-pound fresh, whole, free-range or organic chicken

1 T garlic, about three cloves, chopped

1 lemon, cut thinly into six slices

2 branches fresh rosemary or 2 tsp dried

1 T fresh thyme or 1 tsp dried

1 T sage

1 tsp sea salt

Cracked pepper

2 T olive oil

1 tsp each of three different Indian spices: I use a combination of turmeric, crushed red chili peppers, and 2 tsp ground coriander seed. (To grind coriander, pour dried seed into coffee grinder until the consistency of powder.)

Preheat oven to 375 degrees. Wash and dry chicken. Sprinkle the cavity with a little salt. Combine spices, herbs, garlic, sea salt, and cracked pepper in a bowl and mix together with your fingers.

Gently loosen the breast skin by running your fingers between the skin and the breast meat. Insert three lemon slices on both sides between the skin and the meat. Rub the skin with the herb mixture. Drizzle olive oil over the chicken.

Roast for 70 minutes, or until a leg feels loose when moved. Remove chicken from the oven and place on platter. Skim any fat from the cooking juices and reserve.

Remove skin from chicken; and carve the bird into six pieces. Reheat the cooking juices and pour over chicken pieces. Serves four.

For a few years after we were married, I continued cooking—first establishing a catering business, followed by a Bed & Breakfast in a 100-year old log house Mike and I restored on our property. I hosted a cooking show, *Cooking with Panache*, a fun, lively, unrehearsed cable production filmed in our Northfield kitchen. Many summer nights, Mike and I sat on our stone deck watching the sun disappear behind the cornfields, amazed at the life we had managed to carve out.

The changes in Mike's personality and physical demeanor—which were the result of an as-yet unknown disease—were gradual, and his symptoms would subside for long periods of time. We thought he'd get better and that whatever was happening would eventually just go away. We learned to live with increasingly difficult symptoms.

Before his diagnosis, Mike and I took advantage of our wide web of social and family support. When Mike was anxious or depressed, I could call on people who knew and cared about him, and they eagerly responded to my requests for a fresh perspective.

Keith, an Australian, poet and English professor at Carleton College, was an especially resourceful friend. He would show up at our house on a moment's notice. Nobody would have identified Keith as a therapist, but he was. He had the ability to quickly assess the situation and transform a hopeless, stressful atmosphere into relaxation and joy. He used every tool at his disposal, from hilarious poetry readings to sessions of Reiki, a form of energy healing that balances the body's energy and encourages peace and harmony.

As discussed earlier, the diagnosis of PD may be delayed for a number of reasons. In Mike's case, his diagnosis was delayed, in part, by denial. In the beginning, he dismissed the thought of any serious illness, believing that his problems were associated with stress, getting older and, later on, depression. It was simply by accident that he found himself in a neurologist's office at the Mayo Clinic. He had gone to the clinic for a general consultation and to schedule a colonoscopy, and was referred to a neurologist. The diagnosis was made after Mike completed a few small-motor hand exercises and walked down the hallway while the doctor observed.

Our first response was relief that he didn't have a brain tumor. We high-fived in the grand hallway of The Mayo Clinic, and the sound of our cheers echoed off the marble walls. Within a few years, however, our relief had turned to confusion and anger. Our lives changed and darkened, resulting in the really tough years, when we avoided serious discussions. Because Mike didn't have the conventional tremors, some of our friends expressed doubts that the diagnosis was accurate or even possible, which enabled Mike to slip back into denial.

When our last child left home for college, I realized another exuberant passion, working with high-risk youth. I began a transition from culinary-related occupations—jobs that kept me close to home—to youth advocacy programs and community organizing.

Soon, my days were occupied with writing grants, supporting troubled teenagers, and serving as a guardian *ad litem*—an advocate for the best interests of children who were involved in court procedures. In addition, I developed and administered prevention and intervention programs for the struggling young people the county identified as "at-risk."

Two years later, the reality of Mike's disease dominated our lives, and I escaped even more by becoming totally enmeshed in a new effort to help found a youth-run center, The Northfield Union of Youth.

The kids raised the money and bought their own building, a rundown, wood-floored, tin-ceilinged storefront in downtown Northfield. They named their building "The Key." They owned it and, with some adult guidance, successfully managed their enterprise. Their mission statement said it all, "To give power and voice to youth, and to create a caring community." In retrospect, it's ironic that *power* and *voice* and a *caring community* were just what Mike needed.

The Key still thrives, and the talented adolescents in Northfield continue to practice and perform their music, make their art, publish their poems, create new programs every year, and learn how to contribute to their community in a productive and mutually respectful way.

I loved my job as Executive Director, because every day at The Key we experienced the joy and power of success. Unlike the disintegrating situation at home, the Key kids and I combined our strengths and talents; we rose up to meet every challenge and reduce all barriers. I could make those kids happy just by showing up—and they all smiled.

It became more difficult to reconcile going home at night to face the fact that I could do nothing to help Mike. Even if he *was* happy, I'd never know it because his facial expression was *masked* because of Parkinson's. His voice and his enthusiasm were like his handwriting: flat-lined.

Over the next few years, I watched Mike walking dejectedly across the yard to his studio. His shoulders slumped sadly forward; every day his head seemed to drop lower on his chest in resignation and defeat. I knew he would enter his studio space, sit on a stool, and stare out the window, waiting for something to happen. We could not predict how quickly his PD would progress—and when I would need to be exclusively available to him. After 7 years of conflicted emotions, the truth was looming: my current career was coming to an end.

Mike's anxiety and depression were persistent, and finally we sought professional counseling with an anger-management specialist. In retrospect, I know that particular choice was critical in helping us comprehend the destruction caused by anger and fear.

During those years of stress and confusion, I had to balance my brain with some physical exertion, so I started taking an aggressive 3½ -mile walk twice a day. As I walked, I counted, but once I'd counted the 3,472 rows of corn, counting alone lost its challenge. I began a kind of meditation: counting my steps by using my fingers as an abacus, counting up to 20 on each finger of my left hand, and recording the 100s on my right hand. Then I'd reverse my hands. By counting my fingers down, then up, and then backward and forward, I could tally 4,000 steps with just my fingers. Then I'd shift to my toes, which took a bit more concentration. This exercise worked so well that I was able to "sort and file"—clarify and prioritize—the pressing issues in my head.

Meditation

▶ The health and wellness benefits of meditation are well supported by research.

▶ Meditation is not a religious practice. It is a natural process that allows the mind and body to relax.

▶ Meditation reduces activation of the sympathetic nervous system, which in turn reduces stress hormones such as adrenaline and cortisol.

▶ The relaxation promoted by meditation can reduce stress, anxiety, depression, negative emotions (such as anger), and chronic pain. It also can improve memory, cognitive processing, and sleep.

▶ There are many simple meditation techniques, such as counting breaths while walking, sitting quietly focusing on an object, visualizing an image, or silently repeating a word or sound called a "mantra."

▶ Benefits can be realized by practicing meditation techniques for short periods of time every day.

After 2 years of walking alone, our friends, Billie Jane and Eric, built a log house in the woods near us. Smelling as fresh as clothes just dried on the line, Billie met me with a hug in the middle of the woods every morning at 7:00 A.M. We not only walked through the woods together, but she stayed for the long haul up the steep hills onto the dirt roads, where it was difficult to walk and talk at the same time. She was there waiting in the woods on the coldest Minnesota mornings and the most humid days of summer. Billie was a wise, compassionate confidante. She was my co-worker, and—if there is such a thing—my soul sister.

Loss and Parkinson's Disease

People with Parkinson's, and those who love and care for them, need to cultivate flexibility.

Receiving a diagnosis of Parkinson's disease (PD) can cause people to change their view of themselves, even to question their self-identity. Part of the reason for this is that PD—regardless of the age of onset—can accelerate many of the losses that most of us will experience eventually as we age and decline in physical function, abilities, and independence. Because of the chronic and degenerative nature of the disease, individuals with PD—and their spouses—may face losses on many levels, over many years.

People with PD report feelings of loss in their interpersonal relationships, social life, social status, bodily functions, future plans, occupation, and enjoyable pursuits such as travel or hobbies. An earlier-than-planned retirement may provide relief from dealing with the demands of a job. However, retirement can also cause ambivalence about losing an important source of self-esteem and personal satisfaction. Unresolved grief resulting from the experience of loss can lead to depression.

In March of 2001, on the drive home from our winter sojourn in Kino Bay, Mexico, Mike and I stopped south of the border in Magdalena for a farewell taco and a Pepsi. This departure was different from previous years. Mike was sullen and discouraged about leaving Kino.

"I can't deal with the Minnesota winters for even one more year," he said. "I'll just die." I knew he meant he'd be more and more discouraged with the stark, cold, dangerously icy conditions, so disheartened by the Minnesota weather that he would give up trying to make his life there work.

We talked it over and decided we would have to leave Minnesota in order to keep Mike's health—both physical and emotional—from deteriorating. One major aspect of moving was leaving my job. When I announced my resignation with regret to the Board of The Northfield Union of Youth, I still could not—would not—articulate the truth: I was leaving because my husband had PD, because he needed me to take care of him.

Instead, as I stood before all those children and adults who had pitched in over the years, I jokingly quipped, "I've accepted a position as *companion* to a gentleman, and the job requires that we leave Northfield." Mike and I had not spent much time talking about how difficult leaving was for me. It would be years later, and in a most unlikely setting when I realized that he *did* get it.

Because of the inherent anxiety accompanying PD, Mike and I gravitated toward fixing what *he* needed, when *he* needed it. He was, after all, the one whose life and health seemed uncertain. His needs were *our* priority. That was understandable. He saw his life possibly cut short, with his last years in a wheelchair, and he did not want to be pushing that chair through a snow bank.

I had doubts and fears about moving. How often will I see my children? How would I earn money? Family caregivers do not create cash flow. Would I find new friends, trusted confidants? Will there be time in my life to continue doing what I love? I needed to work as an advocate. How could I accomplish that? I didn't harbor any false hope that our lives would suddenly be more gracious and fulfilling just because we had relocated to a more agreeable climate. We concurred that if we moved, our new environment would not be a retirement community, so that eliminated Arizona and Florida. We made a list of possibilities.

Mike and I were, in essence, free agents familiar with adapting our skills to evolving conditions. The idea of starting fresh in a warmer climate was intriguing, and maybe a necessary—and even a smart—move, but I still wasn't confident we could pull it off.

Two months later, we flew from Minneapolis to the Pacific Northwest for our anniversary. On a 5-day whirlwind tour, we ate our way through several possible cities where we might decide to move.

Beginning with a plate of soft-shell crabs in Seattle, we continued on to smoked salmon with bread and cheese from Whole Foods in Portland, Oregon, and then east to Bend for slow-cooked shoyu ribs. In Ashland, we ate lamb chops and spring rolls with peanut sauce, mussels on the shore in Yachats, and the best coleslaw ever in Lincoln City. The wood-fired pizza at a microbrewery in Eugene was great—and the Wine Country in Northern California was warm, the lifestyle relaxed, and the cuisine outrageously creative.

We ended our tour of cities on the pier in Bellingham Bay, with a take-out lunch from Fairhaven Fish & Chips. By the end of our journey, we had eliminated every place but one as a possible new home: Bellingham, Washington, where the air was deliciously clear (thanks to thousands of acres of fir trees), and an abundant array of fish and fresh produce was available. It didn't take long for me to realize we had made the right decision.

To Mike, the decision to migrate was not complex; it was a simple case of self-preservation that was as natural as geese flying south in the winter. He had spent most of his life working at home. He wanted desperately to continue making his art in a stimulating aesthetic environment with fewer physical demands. Later, he confessed that he had assumed I would love Bellingham and have no difficulty pursuing the activities I enjoyed in our new location.

At first, Mike was completely focused on leaving Minnesota. Just leaving. "I've moved and left family and friends many times," he said. "I knew what I was getting into."

My reality was quite different; my roots went deep. Besides my job and my walking partner, I was leaving family—three of my four children, my only grandchild, my four sisters and their children, and our entire support team.

Even though I prepared myself for another adventure with Mike, I think I wanted to hear from him that he recognized the complications that could result from our decision. Maybe I wanted a guarantee that I would not be "alone in the woods" in an unfamiliar state.

On a cold frosty morning in October 2001, I stood alone in our Northfield kitchen, surveying the stack of more than 100 packing boxes piled almost to the ceiling. The past 21 years flashed before me, beginning with the happy times when we built everything we needed, like the rock walls around the gardens, and the cherry wood kitchen countertops and window trim that Mike had made from trees in our woods.

At those counters and in front of the six-burner range next to me, I had poached, roasted, and sautéed. I had flipped hash browns, frittatas, and crepes in the air, and afterward, I danced. The irony of leaving the kitchen where I had prepared food for so many years was that I had nothing to eat on the morning we were moving.

The kitchen table and chairs were outside in the moving van. All the dishes, pots, pans, and silverware were packed, all the groceries eaten or given away. Luckily, I had prepared two hard-boiled eggs for the road trip to our new home. To say goodbye to my beloved space, I retrieved my egg from the picnic basket, along with a paring knife, a lemon, a small saltshaker, and my favorite traveling pepper grinder.

On top of the final sheet of paper towel left on the countertop, I peeled off the egg shell and cut the egg in half, noticing with some satisfaction that the yolk was clear bright yellow (no green) and perfectly centered inside the white. Yes! You never really know if the yolk is centered until you rinse it with cold water, peel it, and open it up. "This may be an omen!" I thought.

I squeezed a few drops of lemon juice on the egg yolks and sprinkled a little salt and two good grinds of fragrant pepper on it. Then, with my hands folded in silent prayer, I stood back to look at my last humble meal on that counter, in that house in the kitchen of all kitchens, with so many scents and aromas in the walls, and now with a teetering tower of boxes for background—it was a perfect still life.

How to Hard-Boil an Egg

Place eggs in a saucepan and cover with cold water. Bring water to a boil over medium heat. When water boils, reduce heat and simmer for 10 minutes. Transfer eggs to a bowl and quickly cool under cold water. When completely cooled, peel eggs. The yolks should be bright yellow.

The Food and Magic of Kino

True healing is about more than just a well-functioning body. All aspects of who we are must be addressed: physical, emotional, mental, and spiritual.

The transition from Northfield to Bellingham was made even easier thanks to a simple cottage in a small fishing village on the Sea of Cortez in Kino Bay, Mexico.

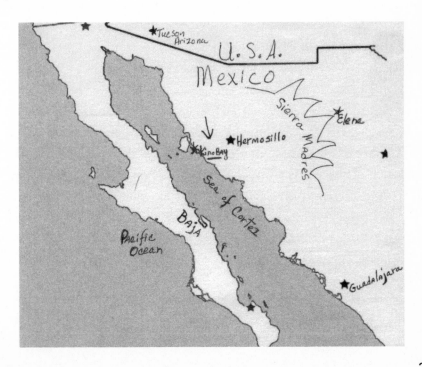

Every year, we spent precious time at our *casita* surrounded by extraordinary characters, a story a day, and new adventures with food. Kino provided immediate warmth and relief from Minnesota winters, and the prevailing stress-free atmosphere of *no problema* and there's always *mañana* brought temporary peace and calm to Mike's anxieties caused by Parkinson's disease (PD).

We continued our visits to Kino after moving to Bellingham, and in Kino we found the treasures that ultimately gave us most of the ingredients we needed for long-term healing.

Everything about our decision to live a portion of each year in Mexico was—as a friend put it—"pushing the envelope." For 14 years, we had taken chances in Mexico, but every risk paid off richly in life lessons and gifts of the spirit.

Years before, when we left Minnesota for our first visit to this small fishing village, we were warned ad nauseam about the lack of "safe" groceries, potable water, and reliable electricity.

"Don't buy anything at the local shops," our well-meaning friends warned. Another friend cautioned, "Be sure to stay away from fresh fruits and vegetables." The myth was that all of the local vegetables were tainted by an unsanitary water supply and poor farming practices. In fact, Kino Bay has its own fresh water well out in the desert.

"Careful of the fish, especially the oysters," one local said. "You'll get sick for certain." So, that first year, just to be safe, we stocked up on canned green beans and asparagus, soups, cocktail wieners, spaghetti, and breakfast cereal—all of which quarreled with my better instincts and culinary desires.

Another frequent traveler to Mexico suggested that we buy our fresh vegetables, chickens, and eggs in Tucson, Arizona, a 6-hour drive from Kino in 90-degree heat. After one heroic but disastrous (now amusing) effort involving an extended stop at the border, spoiled meat, wilted vegetables, and sour milk, we realized that long-distance shopping was not the solution.

Ah well. The next year and every year afterward, we went "South of the Border" with not much more than our candles, books, a sharp knife, lemon zester, and my pepper grinder. The local food supplies in Kino Bay were more than ample—they were luxurious and fresh.

After 14 years of eating our meals on the beach, we are forever imbued with the tastes, sounds, and scents unique to Kino and the fires that feed and warm the people there.

If authenticity is the basis of any good meal, try adding three humble but perfect ingredients: years of practice, an abundance of genuine love of food, and a pound of joy in its presentation. The result would be a close relative to the most memorable meal I have ever eaten anywhere, albeit served in a most unlikely setting. The events that followed opened our eyes and our hearts to the promise and power of hope.

THE COOK, THE HEALER, AND THE DOLPHINS

The sun rises over the Sea of Cortez just east of our *casita* in the small fishing village of Kino Viejo (Old Kino). During the 14 winters we've spent in Kino, I have walked the beach each morning on the damp sand. The air is best early in the morning before the odors of coffee or bacon, toasting tacos, or fabric softener begin circulating and overcome the authentic smells of Kino Bay. The salt washes over last night's nicely cleaned fish skeletons as they loll in and out on the waves. The smoke from the ironwood fires of the wood carvers in Old Kino floats from east to west over the beach, dispensing that defining aroma that brings us back year after year.

Moving to the rhythm of the clanging bells from distant shrimp boats on the horizon, I often looked across the water at Pelican Island. This spot on the beach had the potential for magic. If the sun was just right, the water just warm enough, with no wind at all, there was a chance, a hope, for a view that I've seen only twice—the antics of juvenile, dancing dolphins.

As I returned home from one of my walks, I saw our neighbor, Ramon, holding his long-ashed Boots cigarette out over the deck, while his dog Pepito peed on one of our palm trees.

"I was just telling Mike about a woman I heard of," he said. "A Healer named Elena. She lives up in the mountains." Ramon talked excitedly in his

Castilian accent with heavy overtones of Chicago, where he had spent 20 years of his working life after leaving Chile. He wanted Mike to help him find the Healer. Ramon can charm anybody into doing the nearly impossible.

Ramon's wife, Lola, suffered enormous pain from a rare nerve disorder that affected the right side of her face. The most gentle breeze on the warmest day would force Lola to her bed, where she spent most of her days holding her linen handkerchief up to her face. She had scarcely been out of the house for months.

Ramon had tried everything to ease the pain—marijuana, surgery, Holy Communion, even morphine. Nothing worked.

"Jesus Christ, right?" Ramon pleaded. "Why not try it? Besides," he added, "my back is killing me. Maybe a Healer could help me, too."

Mike laughed. "Yah, and she could take a shot at my Parkinson's. Wouldn't that be something to write home about?"

Mike agreed to drive the Lincoln Continental through the desert and up into the Sierra Madres, and even though I had numerous reservations I agreed to go along.

The next morning, Ramon guided Lola to the Lincoln. It was 75 degrees but she was wearing a silk blouse and a long wool skirt with a heavy sweater that pulled her thin shoulders in and down. A gold scarf was wrapped twice around her tiny neck, and she was holding her lace and linen hankie up tight to her right check. Ramon gently helped her into the back seat, covering her lap and legs with a wool blanket. We waited for our driver. At last, Mike arrived, getting into the car, very gingerly because his back hurt from chopping wood. In addition, just that morning he developed a serious case of *tourista* (diarrhea).

Mike drove that huge boat of a car 25 miles an hour straight up the washed-out sides of mountains, stopping at every available *baño* (bathroom) along the way. The *peligroso* (DANGER) signs appeared around every hairpin turn. It was chillingly clear that two vehicles could not meet without one or both going over the edge. If an oncoming car or truck hit us, how far would we drop? I looked and couldn't see the bottom of the canyon. Twice the gravel shifted under the tires, and I thought we were going over.

After several hours, Ramon pointed out the front window at a restaurant where we might have lunch. "There! Right there," he said, indicating a bombed out, three-sided building with bars on most of the windows.

Deciding this might be the day I died from food poisoning or a car crash, I gave it up to the Lord!

The building turned out to be someone's house—not a restaurant—a dirt-floored house including a living room with a sofa and a blanket on the floor. There was a dusty statue of The Blessed Virgin Mary of Guadalupe across the room. The barefoot virgin stood on a bed of silk violets inside a cut-out plastic 7-Up bottle.

Lola soldiered forward, dragging her wool blanket on the ground across the dirt floor and moaning with every step. Approaching the 7-Up Virgin Mary, she mumbled her first words of the day, "*Ah bueno.*"

As if by magic, a table for four materialized on top of the dusty blanket lying on the floor, along with four placemats, four paper napkins, and four old wooden chairs. A woman appeared and spoke *rapido* Spanish with Ramon.

He translated, lifting his eyebrows as he spoke, "She says she is going to make *special* food for us, not the usual."

A few minutes later, I was transfixed by the plate the woman set in front of me: one fresh warm flour *tortilla grande* folded gently, just so, along the rim and into the center of a white, chipped, stoneware plate. The edges of the tortilla met a perfect circle of Mexican-green puree and a separate pool of Mexican-red puree. The presentation was simply stunning. The tastes were pure essence, separate and combined. The tortilla must have been stretched, thrown, and caught on the woman's elbow at the moment we entered the house. The texture was soft and elastic, with the perfect amount of substance and toasted edges to scoop the purees.

"We grow spinach and tomatoes behind the building," she said in Spanish.

She had combined the reddest, sweetest tomatoes with a subtle burst of fresh basil—but not enough to distract from the color. I think she must have squeezed those vegetables through a sieve as fine as a nylon stocking; they were exquisitely smooth and silken on my tongue.

After lunch and a brief rest and a *baño* stop for Mike, we thanked the cook for the wonderful meal and left to continue our search for the Healer, Elena.

Elena's village was at the peak of a steep, narrow, winding road—it almost teetered at the top of the mountain. There were no cars on the vaguely defined trails that meandered through the ancient compound—that is, except our Lincoln. Dirt paths led to the houses, where bare spots of earth designated the entrances. Most of the homes were constructed of tarpaper and tin; not many were made of *concreto*. Chickens, goats, cats, and dogs, and even cattle, roamed freely on the land. At the gate of the village, we stopped at the Catholic Church and Ramon asked a man where Elena lived. It was just a short distance away.

Tied to a tall shrub outside Elena's house was a *burro*, saddled with an old blanket and ready for duty. Smells of vegetables and herbs stewing engulfed us as we entered a wide courtyard in Elena's compound. She appeared, barefoot and dressed in layers of faded earth-toned fabric; she had strong, square hands, the sign of a serious gardener. Judging by her eyes, she might have been 50 years old, but her skin, the pale amber color of the village soil, made her appear much older. Still, she approached us with strength and serenity, as if she knew we were coming. She walked immediately to Lola, took her tiny face in her hands, and led Lola into the house.

Elena was either a shaman or *curandera*, a Mexican folk healer. *Curanderas* are highly religious; some heal with herbs, some do hands-on spiritual/energy healing, and some manipulate the bones and muscles of the body.

An hour later, we were waiting by the car in bright sunshine when Lola appeared in Elena's doorway without her blanket and with her handkerchief neatly tucked into the pocket of her silk blouse.

Lola spoke more clearly than she had in 3 years. "I feel great," she said with a smile on her face. "*Bueño*, I think I am cured."

Next, it was Ramon's turn, and he followed Elena into the house. Thirty minutes later he emerged, claiming he had no more pain in his back. Mike was buoyant with hope as Elena signaled for him to enter the house. I followed as we passed through Elena's kitchen, where onion skins and cabbage leaves were strewn on the floor and chickens clucked around our feet picking at the fresh scraps of food, typical signs of a Mexican healer. Past the kitchen into a garden of blossoming lemon trees, Elena led us to a small dark room with a single cot. Mike removed his shirt and indicated a scar on his back. Elena pulled a dark bandana over her nose and mouth to protect her from "outside" germs. We did not speak. Elena leaned over the cot where Mike was lying and placed her hands on his back, pressing down on the area he had indicated and then instinctively moved her hands to cover his ears and held both sides of his head. With her eyes closed, she lifted her face toward the ceiling and quietly chanted a prayer.

When Elena left the room, I whispered to Mike, "Well, did you feel anything? What happened?" Slowly, Mike pulled his shirt on and buttoned it. He seemed dazed. "I did feel something, but I couldn't tell you what it was."

Once settled in the Lincoln, Lola made the most amazing suggestion. "Mike, why don't we take the shortcut home? I'll direct you, and we can stop at the restaurant on the freeway, right before the toll booth." Wow! If Lola knew about a shortcut, she couldn't have told us before because it was too painful to speak. Ramon grinned proudly, sitting straight and high in the seat ahead of us. "Yah, Mon, my back feels great too."

We will probably never know the extent of what happened in Elena's small dark rooms, but when we returned to Kino at midnight, Mike's *tourista* and back pain were completely gone and he went peacefully to sleep.

Looking out the window at the end of our bed back in Kino, I saw the lights of the shrimp boats twinkling beyond Pelican Island. I heard their bells and wondered if Elena the Healer really did have curing powers. I closed my eyes knowing that I had left our village with three sick people I loved and had come home with something quite different, something mysterious and hopeful. The mystery began in the restaurant that didn't appear to be a restaurant and continued through three experiences of healing—each on a different level.

True healing is about more than just a well-functioning body. All aspects of who we are must be addressed: physical, emotional, mental, and spiritual.

My own healing began that night with a magical dream, starring a frog as the magician, juggling vegetables in an amphitheater made of grass, which symbolized renewal, regeneration with the fruits of the land.

The next morning, Mike bounced out of bed with enthusiasm for beginning a new sculpture project—the yellow birds for Parkinson's. Standing on the deck, under a palm tree, sipping his tea, he smiled across the sea all the way to the Baja. "Feels like a dream, just to sleep all night with no pain. I hate to jinx it, but whatever Elena did, my body feels transformed. Hard to tell if the power is in the believing, you know—in the hope of a cure."

With Mike's question about healing power on my mind, I walked down the eight steps to the gate and headed east into the brilliant sunrise and pure scents of Kino. For the first time in years, Ramon and Lola stood together at their gate by the sea and waved. Farther down the beach, as I passed Pelican Island, I stopped breathless in my tracks to witness the rare sight of dozens of young dolphins in front of me, diving and flipping, snorting and squealing, dancing on the warmth of the sea and swimming toward the ironwood fires of Old Kino.

> *The key to healing is the ability to focus emotion and energy in our bodies or that of a loved one in a non-invasive and compassionate way.*
>
> *The Divine Matrix by Gregg Braden*

Tortillas with Red and Green Purees

Although I've tried, I just cannot duplicate the magic of that meal in the Sierra Madres. There's a lesson here: Some moments are meant to be appreciated when and where they naturally occur. I humbly offer this close facsimile.

2 *tortillas grande* (large flour tortillas)
4 medium red sweet tomatoes

12 ounces of fresh spinach, washed and with stems removed
2 small leaves of fresh basil

In a medium skillet, add 4 T water and spinach, cook spinach until soft. Place spinach and liquid into a food processor, fitted with metal blade. Puree until smooth. Transfer spinach to a fine sieve. Strain and pour onto two plates making little pools.

Roast the tomatoes in a 400 degree oven for 15 minutes. Peel tomatoes and transfer to the food processor with basil and puree. Strain tomatoes and reheat. Pour pools of tomato puree beside the spinach.

Toast the tortillas by setting them, one at a time, directly on a high burner; gas is easier and quicker, but electric will work too. Just toast the edges, about 10 seconds, and turn over, toast the other side. Fold tortilla along the side of the plate. Serves two.

Healing in Bellingham

We have the ability to heal ourselves and make our dreams a reality. As part of our intention to self-heal, we can create a physical environment to live in that supports and protects us.

A twentieth-century visionary, known simply as "Neville," suggests in *The Divine Matrix*, "We must 'abandon' ourselves to the new possibility and in our love for that state . . . live in the new state and no more in the old." Neville believed that all we experience—literally everything that happens *to* us or is done *by* us—is the product of our consciousness and absolutely nothing else. Our ability to apply this understanding, using the power of our imagination, is all that prevents us from creating miracles in our lives.

The power to heal is something that lives within each of us. But healing takes time—it takes hope, flexibility, and a willingness to consciously change our attitudes and lifestyle. Einstein said, "We can't solve a problem while we're in the same level of thinking that created the problem."

The atmosphere of Kino, and the energy and compassion of Elena, invited us to hope, and therefore recognize the possibilities of looking beyond, making the effort to transcend the disease, and take action to replace our Parkinson's disease (PD) reality with a process of healing.

The risks we've taken by literally *moving to a new state* paid off well! We took a chance when we left Minnesota to live in the more temperate climate of the

Pacific Northwest, but our senses are deliciously rewarded every day. Mike told a friend that moving to Bellingham was our best decision, and I agree, for more reasons than the profusion of seafood and mild Pacific breezes. Parkinson's disease will always travel with us, but we've learned how to politely ask it to move to the back seat so we can see the road ahead.

We designed and built our Bellingham house to accommodate our present needs and the possible future stages of PD. We were determined to incorporate an inspiring and comfortable home environment and a color palette that would sustain us through our transition and the predicted rainy winters of Western Washington.

At first glance, you can't tell that the entrance to our house and the plantings of lavender, germander, and thyme—with their healing hues of purple and violet—are intentionally arranged around a gradual ramp that connects to two porches and two entry doors.

All the doorways inside and out are wheelchair-accessible, and the interior spaces are open to limit the potential of Mike's freezing and falling, two hazards of PD. Our kitchen is invigorating and comforting, with sparkling stainless steel countertops, a Viking range, and refrigerator—vibrant warm colors grace the walls and sturdy timbers lend strength and support.

Mike is a good and happy patient; he follows the advice of doctors and other specialists, with the exception of medications. Since 1993, he has stubbornly (and wisely, as it turns out) chosen to take the lowest possible effective dose of Sinemet®, which is less than half of what the doctor originally prescribed 17 years ago. Mike believes this decision is one of the keys to his slow progression through the stages of Parkinson's. In 2010, his Bellingham neurologist declared him a "model patient."

Neuroprotection: Exercise to Protect Dopamine-Producing Nerve Cells

People living with Parkinson's and caregivers need to follow a regular exercise program and receive support and encouragement from those around them.

Exercise is important for everyone, but especially for people with Parkinson's disease (PD), because it can help improve mobility. Exercise will not stop the disease from progressing, but it can improve strength, so the person with PD doesn't feel powerless and disabled. Exercise also improves emotional well-being. Research indicates that exercise combined with proper diet can lower stress and help us live longer!

Neuroprotection is the term given to mechanisms within the central nervous system that protect neurons from degeneration or death. In the case of PD, neuroprotection refers to protecting dopamine-producing cells from damage.

Preliminary evidence suggests that exercise may provide such neuroprotection. For example, in a study of individuals with PD by Jay L. Alberts, Ph.D., and colleagues at the Cleveland Clinic, motor function improved nearly 35 percent after 8 weeks of tandem bicycle riding, as measured using the Unified Parkinson's Disease Rating Scale. The tandem was used to help the individuals pedal at a greater rate than they could achieve on their own. This is referred to as *forced exercise*. In contrast, *voluntary exercise* performed by individuals in the study—who pedaled at their preferred rate—did not improve PD symptoms. Interestingly, the motor function improvements in the forced exercise group lasted for several weeks after stopping the exercise. They also showed improvements in rigidity and bradykinesia.

Animal studies have shown that exercise appears to have neuroprotective qualities. In rodents, the rate and intensity of the exercise appear to be critical factors if neuroprotection is to occur, as with treadmill running in humans. Studies in non-human primates (monkeys) also suggest that aerobic exercise may have a neuroprotective effect.

At this point, no scientific data exist to recommend one specific exercise over another. Experts recommend finding a type of exercise you enjoy, and have your spouse or a friend join you for encouragement.

Before moving to Bellingham, Mike adamantly refused to participate in formal exercise—even as much as taking a walk down the driveway in Northfield. Now, he admits that for years he invented any excuse—from mosquitoes to slippery ice—to avoid walking any farther than his studio. Beyond 100 feet, he preferred to drive. However, Mike's work as an artist always included strenuous physical activity: building brick kilns, wedging clay, throwing and trimming huge pots on the wheel, loading and unloading the kiln, and later wrestling with panels of steel—cutting, shaping, and welding.

Since 2005, Mike has religiously attended yoga classes 2 days a week. As a result, his strength and balance, breathing, and overall sense of hope are better tuned than they would be without yoga. He is so committed to his yoga schedule that, after a middle-of-the-night fall during which he cracked a rib, he drove all the way to town to tell Abby, his instructor, that he couldn't participate. Equally dedicated to her students, Abby offered to give Mike private lessons with an individualized program until he fully recovered.

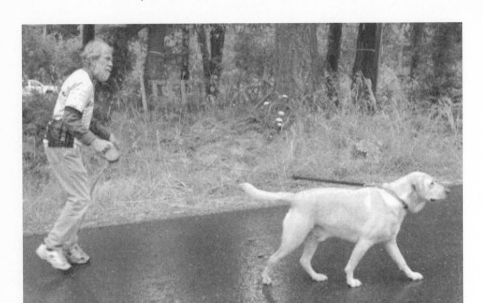

Besides his strict attention to rigorous yoga, Mike and our yellow lab/ retriever, Rueben, walk 1 mile every morning, drizzle or shine. Straining at the leash 3 feet ahead of Mike, Rueben pulls him up the driveway, and then helps him tackle the steep lane to the main road. After one more gradual incline, they turn around and head effortlessly down the hill toward home.

Without Rueben's help, Mike leans too far forward and has some difficulty making it up the hill. Once he told me, "If the hill was any steeper, I'd have to install a wheel on my nose." He anticipates his morning walk, and it's as habitual as his winter breakfast of oatmeal with a handful of raisins and sprinkling of dried sour cherries.

Since we moved to Bellingham, I have continued my walking/counting method of mental relaxation every day, and enjoy a breathtaking route alongside Douglas firs, big leaf and vine maples, native *Heuchera* and salmon berries, blackberries, wild strawberries, and ferns.

From our house, up three moderate inclines, I pass happily through a dozen stimulating olfactory zones of fresh clear air, to the silent shore of a majestic mountain lake and back home again—4,720 steps. It truly clears the debris in my head, and nobody's locked me up yet!

Besides the importance of daily exercise, extensive research has shown that a support network is critical to the healthy survival of those who care for the sick or elderly. An ideal support team usually includes family, friends, and neighbors, each making a unique contribution.

Together, Mike and I have seven children. His three, Randy, Greta, and Jon, range in age from 53 to 43, and my four, Sean, Geoffrey, Andrew, and Sarah Anne, are 39 to 43. Nine of my ten grandchildren have been born since we moved to Bellingham, most of them in Minnesota.

On a daily basis, we are grateful for the gift of having a child living just 7 miles away. My son, Andy, and his wife, Juliana, moved to Bellingham from California 2 years after we did. Andy is a teacher and Juliana, also a teacher, stays home with their three young children.

Besides the built-in moral and physical support provided by Andy and Juliana, the grandchildren add profound joy to our lives. They don't notice anything different about Mike. They sit on his lap and listen as he plays the harmonica. They love him unconditionally and treat him as if he's normal, and that makes him smile. Our other children and grandchildren visit in person or by phone or e-mail on a regular basis.

As a caregiver, I value the ability to stay in contact with people who know and care about both Mike and me. It's helpful and comforting when someone offers to "come take Mike for a ride."

For example, last year Mike's friend Skip came from Minnesota for a 2-week visit. Mike and Skip have been car-buddies for over 40 years. As it turned out, while he was here, I had to go back to Minnesota to help my daughter, who was sick. Skip stayed with Mike while I was gone, helped him repair his Dodge, and made sure he was safe, fed, and entertained. We did not plan it that way, but it was a lovely bit of synchronicity.

The cautions of Agnes, a long-time friend and caregiver, remind me of the potential pitfalls that may be encountered with well-meaning offers of assistance. Agnes's husband had Alzheimer's, and her children and grandchildren lived in another state. She wanted desperately to be involved with her young grandchildren but was convinced she couldn't. She made two memorable observations: One, "Toddlers and Alzheimer's don't mix," and, "Usually well-intended people coming to help results in *more* work rather than less." Agnes's strategy was to ignore her needs, shut her eyes, plow through, and hope for the best.

Perhaps a better answer would be to encourage the kind of help Skip provided. He not only helped rebuild the Dodge, he literally came from another state and "took Mike for a ride."

Another good example of support occurred the year Mike was invited to attend the Morris Udall awards dinner hosted by the Michael J. Fox Foundation. The dinner was staged at Tiffany's in New York, and was designed to honor Team Fox members who have made contributions to PD research. I could not attend the dinner, but I asked Mike's sister, Karin, if she would make the cross-country trip with him. She took loving care of her brother, and she also created a scrapbook of the entire weekend. These generous acts remind us of the meaning of compassion.

Our life in the Great Northwest offers other benefits besides the obvious one of having access to fresh Pacific salmon. The Northwest Parkinson's Foundation (NWPF) is headquartered in Seattle. Inspired by the work of Bill Bell, the Executive Director, and his small but efficient staff, NWPF reinforces the power of hope. Our efforts to help NWPF raise money for PD education and quality of life are encouraged, enthusiastically recognized, and genuinely appreciated. We have met other people with PD, who share their stories of challenge, downright courage, and triumph. Every day, we have the opportunity to witness mercy and grace within this community of people with PD, their caregivers, and medical professionals. We have also been blessed with smart, compassionate friends, colleagues, and attentive caring neighbors—we hold each person gently and dearly.

I was also fortunate to meet Dr. Nanette Davis and assist her in her research project focused on women caring for their sick and elderly loved ones. Through the process of our discussions on caregiving, I was finally freed to admit out loud my own emerging role as a caregiver. Prior to meeting Nanette, Mike objected to my being described as a "caregiver," primarily because he would then be forced to admit he needed care. He disapproved of caregiver support groups and even support groups to help him. As I worked with Nanette, my situation crystallized: I was indeed a caregiver. The truth hung on as I drove home after each work session and, within weeks, I announced my role. This acceptance helped move Mike and me toward a clearer and more constant communication about our everyday needs and responsibilities toward each other. At last, Mike acknowledged the difficult truth: he needed care.

Nanette's friendship also opened my eyes to the possibilities of living well with PD. When, at last, I verbalized that I was a caregiver, I began to recognize the seemingly random acts of kindness that had been occurring all along, given to us by people who were now our Bellingham support team.

Reciprocity

*One compassionate deed properly acknowledged surely
leads to another.*

Anonymous

*A*cross the Street is a short nonfiction story written by Bia Lowe. The author watches from her window over time as her sick elderly neighbor progresses through the final stages of a fatal disease. "He began to study his feet as he walked," Lowe wrote, "and I watched his steps grow smaller. Eventually he had to rely on a cane, and that soon gave way to a walker."

This story could have been told by our young neighbor, Pat, a part-time fireman and stay-at-home dad. Pat's kitchen window is situated so that he can see Mike in places where I can't—making his way out to his studio, stacking firewood by the garage, or mowing the lawn.

Pat didn't know it, but from *my* vantage point, I could see *him* looking into our yard one rainy winter day. Soon afterward, Mike came in the house scared, wet, and exhausted. He told me he was having a hell of a time lifting the firewood into the wheelbarrow, but he kept trying and kept dropping the logs. He was afraid he'd fall on the concrete. Before anything dangerous happened, as if by accident, Pat appeared at Mike's side.

"Well, as long as I'm here," Pat offered nonchalantly, "I could help load that?" He delivered the fully loaded wheelbarrow to our back door, made sure Mike got inside, and then disappeared into his own yard.

The author of *Across the Street* asks herself, "And what of me? Is there a vantage point, say, from a neighbor's window, where my descent can be witnessed? . . . If my number's up and something has begun to grow inside me, and I can't stand or walk even an inch without someone at my side, will there be someone who loves me, come to take me out in the world for a ride. . .?"

Later, I asked Pat about that day by the woodpile. I told him I had observed *his* observance, and that what he did for Mike was an awe-inspiring act of kindness.

"Just paying attention," he said, dropping off our recycle containers that he'd fetched from the road above the house.

Pat is compassionate and smart. He never interferes with Mike's actual abilities, but he gets there just in time. His presence in our lives is invaluable.

With reciprocity in mind, we continue to build our network carefully, one relationship at a time. I've also learned that meaningful, short, in-person visits and phone conversations with my Minnesota sons, Sean and Geoffrey, and my sisters are sustaining. We don't waste much time on idle or negative chatter, but we are generous with the phrase, "I love you," and we try harder to *just pay attention.*

Women who are caregivers, and who are fortunate enough to have supportive daughters, cope better emotionally over the long haul of caregiving. I am fortunate. My daughter Sarah and I laugh and cry together; share our dreams; and cook and tend to babies with a matching spirit of love and care. Sarah and her brothers have witnessed and participated in every step of my cooking and caregiving careers, and—as adults and parents—they embrace the process of cooking good food with great joy and celebration.

Seeds of Nurturing

*Mastering the fine art of cooking delicious, nutritious food
for health will help you to feel more in control of
Parkinson's disease.*

When I was 2½ years old, Grandma White boosted me up to the kitchen table on top of the Minneapolis phone book and tied me to the back of the chair with a dish towel. I watched as she kneaded bread dough, and I was so close to the action (she later told me) that my entire head was dusted in white.

With a new baby about to be born, my mother was in the hospital. Grandma packed her multicolored patchwork leather handbag with her prayer book and rosary, her St. Francis holy cards, several packets of yeast, her biggest wooden spoon, and a rolling pin, and she came to stay with us until mother and baby returned home.

Baking was Grandma's method of preparing the atmosphere and preventing—as best she could—any loneliness or confusion that might occur during the absence of our mother and the pending transition to life with a new baby.

With my chin on the table, I was entranced by her hands in the dough, as she skillfully punched, folded, and turned the gooey mass, magically transforming it into a smooth, silken mound. Grandma was a baker, and Parker House rolls topped by three precise mini-knobs were her specialty. Her purpose was to fill our house with the sweet scents of love and care. The aroma of baking, roasting, or sautéing fresh ingredients still calms my soul and grounds me to the place where I'm cooking. Through all the stages of Parkinson's disease (PD), food has been my most effective tool in the quest to create an atmosphere of optimism and anticipation for whatever is coming next.

THE SANDWICH EXTRAORDINAIRE

In food preparation, details are important and result in appreciation and satisfaction; the nurturing *is* in the details. My first opportunity to practice my grandmother's style of nurturing took place late on a snowy afternoon, New Year's Day, in the year that I was 12. I sat warming my feet by the fire in the living room. Across the room on the sofa, my father rested with a book. He was drifting off to sleep, tired from a long day. After our traditional early dinner, my mother and all eight children had followed my father to the river, where he had shoveled an ice rink for skating and built a bonfire on the shore to warm us.

But now, everyone was napping except me, and I was hungry! I imagined my father must be hungry, too. The memory of dinner leftovers made me ravenous. I could still smell the roast beef with the crispy edges all rubbed with salt, cracked pepper, and chunky garlic.

Watching the embers in the fireplace, I imagined what I could do with that meat. I looked across the room at my father. "How would you like a sandwich?" I asked.

From behind his book, he mumbled, "You bet. That sounds fine." I could tell from his response that he wasn't inspired by what I might accomplish in the kitchen—and for good reason. Up until to that moment, I had never cooked anything by myself, and I'd never used a sharp knife.

My first adventure was to discover exactly what was in the refrigerator. Besides the roast, I chose a tomato, a big white onion, two lettuce leaves, fresh parsley, and a container of mayonnaise that my mother had made the day before.

I cut two slices of Grandma's bread, trying to keep the serrated knife straight and the bread even and thin, but not flimsy. Then, it was on to the beef, which I carefully cut in one round thin slice, clean and straight. Feeling more confident with the knife, I sliced four rounds of tomato, peeled the onion, and carefully planed two paper-thin onion wafers.

I spread one slice of bread with a bare coating of butter and a thin sheet of mayonnaise on the other slice—all the way to the edges. Placing a ruffled lettuce leaf, just so, over the mayonnaise, I sprinkled parsley over the lettuce, folded the meat carefully over the tomatoes and arranged the onion slices on top. The ruffle of lettuce showed just slightly around the outside edge of the sandwich with a simple elegance that made me feel proud.

My father set his book down, sat up, and surveyed the tray holding his sandwich.

"Hmmm," was the only sound he made as I backed up toward the fireplace. It seemed like it took him forever to eat that sandwich. Finally, he was finished. He wiped his hands, folded the napkin, and placed it back on the tray.

Then, as if he had no concept of the power of his next words, he looked across the room right into my eyes and said, "That, young lady, was not just a sandwich. *That* was an experience." At that moment, I forgot that I'd been starving earlier. I felt completely full. I did not need a sandwich after all, because the *experience* of nurturing someone else was nurturing for me, too.

Through her life and even her death, Simone Beck influenced my dedication to good food, and the understanding that just because a person is sick does not mean they have to settle for uninspired cuisine.

Cooking has remained a joyful and sustaining endeavor through various careers and chapters of my life. By the time I was 29, I was co-owner of the

Palette & Wheel and operated the cafe at The Minnetonka Art Center. Two years later, we added the restaurant at The Walker Art Center in Minneapolis.

From 1977 to 1980, while I was still running the Art Center's cafe, I had the rare opportunity to study and travel with the Grand Dame of French cooking, the legendary Simone "Simca" Beck, famous mentor to Julia Child and co-author of two volumes of *Mastering the Art of French Cooking*.

Simca's cookbooks changed the attitudes of American cooks and, as a result, cooking became a worthwhile and respectable pursuit for home cooks as well as professional chefs.

As stated by the authors in the Foreword of *Mastering the Art*: "The excellence of French cooking, and of good cooking in general, is due more to cooking techniques than to anything else." The trick is to apply the fundamental techniques and always use good basic ingredients.

Simca's lessons are still relevant today; they have transcended all cooking fads, fusions, and pretensions. She encouraged—actually, she demanded—a conscious style of living. She taught me more about cooking than how to make sauces and mousses, soufflés and pates; she exposed me to the French attitude about food and life. Every ingredient, from a humble pea to the plumpest chicken, is respected and has a purpose, both aesthetically and nutritionally.

"After a while," Simca wrote, "you won't need to follow a recipe. You will open the refrigerator, see what is available, and create. You will begin to sense when there is a missing ingredient, and you will know exactly what that ingredient is."

In 1977, the year after my first classes with Simca at L'Ecole des Trois Gourmandes, in Bramafam, Provence, she invited me to accompany her to Bourbonne-les-Bains, a hydrotherapy spa in the Haute Marne area of eastern France, where Simca took the "cure" for 3 weeks every spring. When she learned that I had undergone back surgery, she decided I should join her at Bourbonne-les-Bains.

I learned important lessons about cooking and eating during the road trip from Bramafam to the spa with Simca and her husband Jean. We stopped for roadside picnics of simple sandwiches made with pure fresh local butter and thin slices of locally cured ham. Every bite was *an experience* reminiscent of my father's appreciative declaration when I was 12.

Simca, Jean, and I also enjoyed dinners at three-star restaurants. The chefs knew (and undoubtedly feared) Simca because she was a Michelin judge. We drove into Switzerland to the famous Hotel Crissier and luxuriated in a dinner prepared by a nervous up-and-coming chef, Freddie Girardier, who was anxious to earn his final star. Standing next to our table, he looked surprised as Simca questioned him about his reasons for undercooking the four tiny peas in the *scallops en croute*!

We also visited a small quiet French country inn, arriving mid-morning. It wasn't the food that impressed me, so much as Simca's audacious entrance into the restaurant. The sign on the door said, "Closed" and "Lunch will be served at noon." While Jean and I turned to go back to the car, Simca rang the bell and waited for the proprietor to open the door. The owner appeared and Simca requested lunch. A discussion in French ensued, and finally the woman acquiesced and opened the door for us to enter.

Jean and I trotted obediently behind as Simca marched straight ahead into the woman's kitchen and, with her hands planted firmly on her hips, asked the woman to open the refrigerator. I was stunned.

"Let me see what you have," Simca said in mildly agreeable tone, "and I'll tell you what we'd like." After studying the entire contents, Simca pulled out four or five ingredients and placed them on a long wood work table—a wire basket of *oeufs* (eggs), a crockery pot of *moutarde* (mustard), two chunks of *fromage* (cheese), a bundle of greens and a handful of *herbes* (herbs).

Jean and I followed Simca to the inn's empty dining room and sat down to wait for the improvisation of a simple parsley omelet, followed by a green salad tossed in a savory mustard vinaigrette sprinkled with fresh tarragon leaves and served with a local cheese and warm crusty French bread. The following recipe is similar to the one we shared at the Inn.

Green Salad with Parisian Dressing

1 head of red or green Bibb lettuce, washed and spun dry
3 T olive oil
1 tsp Dijon mustard
1 T red wine vinegar
Salt and pepper
1 T fresh herbs (tarragon, parsley, chives, or basil), minced

In a large salad bowl, whisk olive oil and vinegar together until thoroughly combined. Whisk in mustard until smooth. Add herbs, salt and pepper, and whisk again. Pour ¼ cup dressing in bottom of salad bowl and top with washed lettuce. Just before serving, toss the salad. You can store the remainder of the dressing in the fridge, in a tightly covered container. Shake before using.

Once we arrived in Bourbonne-les-Bains and were comfortably settled in our simple lodgings, Simca and I spent many hours reading about food, discussing food, and responding to requests from aspiring cooks (mostly American) hopeful of winning a spot at Simca's cooking school.

In 1991, after months of heart problems, Simca refused to eat the unimaginative diet recommended for her heart health. She died soon afterward at the age of 87. Her cousin reported on the irony of Simca's death in her *New York Times* obituary: "The doctor said that because she wouldn't eat, she died."

It makes sense that someone who cared so passionately about food and its preparation would be disheartened and demoralized by being forced to eat insipid and uninspiring food.

With my own mission of nurturing others with nutritious food in mind, I can still hear Simca say, "That situation should never be allowed." Everyone, including those who are sick and frail, is entitled to healthy food that tastes good.

From the Other Side of the Window

People with Parkinson's disease are easily distracted and have difficulty performing more than one task at a time, or having multiple conversations, but it's best to be patient and wait. This affords them the opportunity to complete the task themselves rather than having someone else step in and "rescue" them.

Summer 2008: With our earphones in place, my youngest sister, Sarah, and I sat in the darkened room at Western Washington University's speech and hearing clinic. We were observing Mike through the one-way glass window. On the other side, the lights were bright as we watched his student therapist, Melinda, a gentle, compassionate young woman, greet Mike with excitement and genuine joy. She introduced him to a visiting student, Nicole, who was going to sit in on Mike's final session at the clinic. He took a chair across the small table from the students.

My sister and her 30-year-old daughter, Caitlin, were visiting Bellingham from Minnesota for 3 days. We planned to observe Mike's class for just a few minutes. We were anxious to get to the grocery store because the fresh Copper River salmon was in and supplies do not last long.

Melinda had been working with Mike for two quarters on speech and swallowing, which are at-risk functions for people with Parkinson's disease (PD). Mike was graduating from the program, and to celebrate his success Melinda had asked him to assemble a portfolio of his artwork to present at this last session. My sister and I watched through the glass as Mike placed the envelope containing his CD and other photos on the table while Melinda opened her laptop. Next to her, Nicole set up a digital meter to measure his voice strength and projection.

"We'll get the background noise going," Melinda explained, as she clicked her mouse and tuned into a radio station on her computer screen. "Then, Mike, you can show us what you brought. Maybe you could explain your artwork, using all the techniques we've worked on. Is that okay?"

After coaching Mike and learning the many nuances of his disease, Melinda had decided to study PD more thoroughly for her graduate studies. She complimented Mike on his hard work and positive attitude while he tried to remove his materials from the envelope.

We could clearly hear the rustling of papers through our earphones, and Mike seemed to have forgotten that Sarah and I were watching him. I noticed that he had difficulty sliding the papers past the sticky flap of the envelope. Mike has limited manual dexterity, which is not related to PD but complicated by it. The condition, *Dupuytren's contracture disorder*, tightens the tendons of his hands and pulls his two little fingers downward into his palms. He was getting one of those fingers stuck on the bottom of the envelope, making it impossible to slide the papers out.

The young women did not compensate for his difficulty with idle conversation or silly excuses as they watched him, and they didn't make any attempts to do it for him. They smiled and calmly waited. I knew he was distracted, impeded by that envelope flap, which threw him off his much anticipated presentation.

As he had admitted the previous week, "Any stress at all tips the first domino," laughing at the inevitability. "Almost anything causes stress, so there you have it."

I held my breath. His brow was furrowed, and his feet and legs began to twitch under the table as he concentrated on releasing the contents of the envelope. Out of necessity, I had begun to read Mike's cues of stress, fatigue, and frustration. The familiar signs of stress appeared, but Mike does not give up, ever. Not on the little things, like sticky envelope flaps. Not on the big things either, like living with PD.

Mike was a better person on that day than he was 10 years ago or even yesterday, and he was proud because this was his graduation day. He was making progress, and the two young students were eagerly and patiently waiting to view his enormous, incredible, life-filled sculptures. I knew he was aware they were waiting. He has learned that patience is *the* archangel of all saintly virtues, and that it works both ways.

Mike finally succeeded in extracting the papers and CD from the envelope, and Melinda slid the CD into the computer. As the young women watched the screen, the radio program continued as competition designed to force Mike to concentrate on volume and articulation so he could be completely understood.

Two weeks before, Melinda had asked if I'd noticed the difference in Mike's speech. I told her we had, and that we used the hints she'd recommended. But Mike said he generally saves his energy for people who have little or no understanding of PD and how the disease affects every part of his body, including his larynx, lungs, and even his tongue.

You couldn't tell by his face, but he *was* happy. Mike is also aware of how his expression, or lack of it, affects other people.

"It's hard enough for people to make eye contact with me," he said, "because I seem to be unaware or apathetic. It's too much to expect someone to wait it out." Mike told me he is very conscious of the moment when his listener begins to lose interest. He can feel it, even in a phone conversation. So, he makes every effort to shorten his stories, or just allow them trail away. "Once I get off-track or begin to pay attention to my own voice," he said, "I'm instantly distracted and forget where I'm going."

Sometimes, it really is laborious for Mike to complete a softly delivered, stuttered, or slurred message, but on that day he worked hard to communicate with the students.

The slideshow began with the sculptures he had created in Northfield years ago and then moved to Bellingham. Melinda and Nicole were clearly intrigued; their eyes were wide and focused on the computer screen.

"Wow! Is that in your yard?" Melinda asked. "Here in Bellingham? It's so huge."

"Yes, that is a sculpture of me and my wife," he told them, squinting at the screen.

As they talked about the sculpture, I recalled a day 20 years before when Mike and his assistant, Todd, installed it by the swimming pool in Northfield. Mike, my children, and I built that pool totally by hand in a rock outcropping down the hill from our house.

We hosted the outdoor sculpture competition sponsored by The Northfield Arts Guild. I catered the event, serving individual picnic baskets with French potato salad, Cornish pasties made with a cream cheese and butter crust filled with carrots, beef tenderloin, celery, and sweet potatoes cooked in an herb and wine sauce. For dessert we prepared individual fresh strawberry tartlets. Inside each basket was a small bouquet of fresh herbs tied to a cloth napkin.

In the studio, Mike and Todd had finished the last weld just seconds before the panel of judges appeared around the corner and awarded them First Prize. Overwhelmed by fatigue, the last-minute finish, and the honor, Mike and Todd jumped in the pool with their clothes on.

As he looked at the slide, Mike was probably recalling the joy and relief of that day too. "We call this one *The Greeters*," he said. "The arch is welded stainless steel, and the couple under the arch is constructed of 20-gauge steel that is meant to age and rust over time. We moved these pieces with us from Minnesota."

"Did you do all the work on that, Mike? How do you get the swirly design on the surface?" Medinda asked.

"With a circular grinder," he said, answering half her question. As they moved through the slideshow of sculptures, Mike answered questions and I watched the voice volume meter in front of Nicole. Mike was doing very well according to the test measurements.

Melinda prodded him to explain the new slide. "Tell us about this one, Mike. That looks so colorful . . . so creative! Who'd think of using bikes that way?"

Mike cleared his throat, a frequent occurrence with PD. "That's a deck railing I built for a youth-run youth center in Northfield." Then, almost as an afterthought, he added, "My wife's project . . . it was on the river. Stolen bikes sometimes end up in the river. I salvaged them, welded them together, and made the railing." I grabbed my sister's hand and stared ahead through the glass. Mike had never mentioned the work I left behind in Minnesota. I thought he didn't recognize or remember the importance of what was accomplished. My sister knew his lack of recognition had been an issue for me.

I could tell Mike wanted to elaborate on the bicycle railing. He began to explain to the students how he used stainless steel tubing to connect the bikes, simulating the waves of the river. It was complicated, though, and his brow furrowed as his voice lost volume. The radio announcer won this round. Mike's voice slipped into the background and he let the story go unfinished, as often happens.

Even though he doesn't talk about it, I think the subject is emotional for him, too. It was clear that the bicycle railing triggered memories of friends and history created over the years in that small town on the river. Mike quietly pondered the photograph on the computer screen, and for an agonizing 2–3 minutes we heard only the voice of the radio announcer. "What is Mike thinking?" I wondered.

Then, still staring at the screen, he cleared his throat again and—with a hint of melancholy in his voice—clarified his earlier statement.

"My wife was the Executive Director. . . . It's The Northfield Union of Youth. . . . It was a big deal . . . still going today."

My sister and I sat silently behind the glass, staring straight ahead, barely breathing as we listened to him and interpreted what he'd said, and what he'd left unsaid. His words and the emotions behind them were my first clue that Mike understood the magnitude of what I had left behind.

Yellow Birds of Hope

*Ways can be found to compensate for the limitations
caused by Parkinson's disease. After 35 years of making
pottery, Mike realized he could no longer wedge clay,
throw pots, and trim and decorate pottery because he no
longer had the necessary small-motor function of his hands.
However, he could successfully work with 8 × 10-foot
sheets of stainless steel, so he turned his creative attention
to building huge welded steel sculptures.*

Twenty-three yellow bird sculptures fly high above the garden on 6-foot stainless steel rods. They represent the hope that someday there will be a cure for PD. The vibrant orange and yellow birds were created by Mike to raise money for the Michael J. Fox Foundation's Parkinson's disease (PD) research, and the Northwest Parkinson's Foundation's program designed to increase the quality of life for people with PD.

When the yellow birds in our garden appeared on the screen, Melinda and Nicole were captivated by the sight. The buoyant height of the birds seemed to lift the spirits on both sides of the therapist's window, reminding us of how much we had gained by living in the atmosphere of Bellingham, with its clean air, panoramic beauty, and web of support. In Bellingham, all things well-planted grow with exuberance.

"Oh those birds! They're so beautiful," Melinda said, "so graceful. How did you come up with that design?"

Mike began the story of our winter getaway in Kino Bay, Mexico, the source of his yellow bird inspiration. I knew he wanted to tell the women about the generosity and compassion of the Mexican welders, Javier, Estephan, and Gordo, who helped him shape and weld a fence of birds between our *casita* and the sea. But he recognized that his energy was running low, and regretfully that story faded into the background.

The seagulls bob on the Sea of Cortez, floating freely, buoyantly with no restrictions and no impediments, unlike the movements of people with PD. Mike had sat in the sand for hours sketching the seagulls.

The student therapists were looking at the photographs of our Bellingham kitchen garden filled with heathers, blooming lavender and thyme, French tarragon, oregano, sage, marjoram, artemisia, roses, and other lush luminaries.

"Oh, what is that flower . . . right there?" Melinda asked, pointing to the garden slide on the screen. Mike looked anguished, wanting desperately to recall the name of the flower in the frame—the tall plant with lime-colored flowers that balloon at the ends of primeval-looking vines snaking over the garden floor. He cleared his throat and studied the screen, haltingly identifying most of the other plants. I felt the dials on my earphone unit, hoping to locate a two-way voice apparatus. I wanted to tap on the window to get his attention and mouth out the word he needs, or better yet, use sign language and gestures to tell him so he wouldn't have to struggle for the word: *You 4 B Ahhhh!* Euphorpia.

At the end of the show, Melinda and Nicole sat back in their chairs and smiled across the table at him. They seemed amazed by what they'd seen, and for a few moments they were speechless.

"You really are an artist, Mike," Melinda said, finally. "Thank you." She asked if he'd be interested in creating something for an auction at the University. He smiled a little as he began the task of putting his CD and drawings back in the envelope with the sticky flap. The entire session seemed to have taken all the concentration and energy he had left—until dinner, that is!

After nourishing our bodies at home with Copper River salmon, smoke-cooked over plum wood and served with a new Napa cabbage slaw recipe featuring sesame oil and seeds, arugula and toasted hazelnuts, we set out to nourish our souls.

Napa Cabbage Slaw with Sweet Corn

This is the best summer slaw when the corn is perfectly fresh.

4 cups Napa cabbage, cut in whole rounds about ¼-inch wide

½ cup arugula, scissor-cut

1 cob of super sweet-white corn, cut raw from the cob

1 T sesame oil

1 T red wine vinegar

¼ cup low-fat mayonnaise

2 tsp fresh lemon juice

4 T toasted hazelnuts, finely chopped

2 tsp toasted sesame seeds

Combine vinegar, sesame oil, lemon juice, and mayonnaise in the bottom of medium-sized salad bowl. Mix to incorporate ingredients. Add cabbage, corn, and arugula. Toss to coat cabbage. Just before serving, top with toasted hazelnuts and sesame seeds. Add salt and cracked pepper to taste. Don't let this sit for over half an hour before serving—it will get watery.

Try other raw vegetables, such as raw grated sweet potato, parsnips, radish root, or jicama, combined with cabbage, or other sturdy leaves such as swiss chard, cut in the chiffon style (½-inch circles). Serves two.

After dinner, Mike organized an event to entertain my sister and her daughter, Caitlin. We drove downtown to the Acoustic Frog Tavern to hear a young musician—Mike's distant cousin—play guitar. We seldom go out after dinner, but we loved every minute of it, and I wondered why we don't do such wonderful things more often. Is it just because it's dark and we're 60 and 70 years old, and Mike has PD?

The next night we had sea scallops with cannellini beans.

Sea Scallops with Cannellini Beans

2 sea scallops (the larger ones)

2 T butter substitute such as Earth Balance or Smart Balance (Earth Balance is dairy-free; if you can't find it, use Smart Balance Free, regular Smart Balance, or a similar product)

½ cup sweet onion, thinly sliced

1 15-ounce can cannellini beans, drained and rinsed

Juice of half a lemon, about 1 T

2 T olive oil

1 T flat parsley, chopped

Salt and freshly cracked pepper

2 T Pesto (Pantry, page 98)

4 T Aioli (Pantry, page 99)

Heat the beans in the microwave for 3 minutes or in a saucepan on the stove over medium heat for 5 minutes. Remove from heat and add lemon juice and 1 T olive oil, parsley, salt, and pepper.

Melt butter substitute in a heavy skillet and, when hot, add onions. Reduce heat and simmer, stirring onions until they begin to caramelize. Add scallops and cook on one side, about 5 minutes. Turn scallops over and cook another 5 minutes. Remove from heat.

Divide beans between two plates. Spoon onions on top of beans. Arrange scallop on top of onions. Drizzle with aioli and highlight with pesto. Serves two.

After dinner, Mike casually suggested we take Sarah and Caitlin to see the new movie at Bellingham's "Art Cinema." The movie, *On a Wing and a Prayer*, was about a Muslim man who was learning to fly in America.

As the movie began, I had no idea it was filmed in Bellingham until I recognized our little International Airport and the main character's office in downtown Bellingham. Mike knew, though. He also knew that at the end of the movie, the stars would appear in person. They were dressed in the same clothes they wore in the movie, the student pilot sporting his white short-sleeved shirt and dress pants, and his wife dressed in the customary long billowing pants and a black and white headscarf.

"We just stopped by to answer questions about being Muslim—and being misunderstood in America," said the man.

"Why would he even try to fly," I wondered, "with all the barriers and stereotyping resulting from 9-11?"

The husband and father of three continued, "We wanted to give you a chance to meet us in person, to understand that we live an ordinary life; we are regular people, and we are also Muslim."

After the movie, on our way to find some gelato, Caitlin piped up from the backseat, "Well, just when I thought things couldn't get any cooler, there they were, the stars, in person—just prancing down the center aisle. You're a stud, Uncle Mike."

Mike is a *cool* guy, proud of his spontaneous acts, and in some ways—like the Muslim student pilot—he knows how it feels to be misunderstood. He'd like people to know that he is a regular guy with a normal life, and that he also has PD.

Mike: Yes, I have felt misunderstood, because of the drunken-appearing way I walk or the soft stammering manner I use to begin a sentence. Sometimes I misrepresent myself, because of my lack of facial expression. I'm sorry for this inconvenience.

A few years ago, after dinner with friends in Minneapolis, we stopped to get gas on our way home. It was 1:00 A.M., and a police car followed us into the gas station. Policemen always make Mike nervous.

The policeman approached our car as Mike was filling the tank. I knew his stress level would rise if a police car came anywhere near his driving privileges.

The policeman inquired, "I've been watching you try to get that hose in the tank. Have you been drinking tonight?"

"No. I'm sorry, Officer," Mike said. "I have Parkinson's disease." The policeman apologized, shook Mike's hand, and wished him good luck. I was surprised and proud of Mike for his forthright no-nonsense response.

During the early stages of PD, Mike was happy to have an "out," an identifiable malady that would explain his appearance. "I let people know it's out of my control," he would tell them. "I don't want anyone to judge my intellect by the imperfection of my mobility or speech."

In 2005, Mike made a solo trip from Bellingham to Washington D.C. to meet President Bush. Mike's son, Randy, was a member of the White House press corps, and he invited Mike to be his guest at the White House Correspondent's Christmas party.

Mike needed serious clothing for this auspicious occasion. He secretly hoped he could find a nice dress shirt, but with no buttons. By this time, he'd begun to dread the task of buttoning his clothes. He desperately wanted to *do it himself*, but when time is an issue stress builds and the fine motor skill of buttoning is even more daunting.

For example, one evening Mike was dressing for the symphony, an event he loves. I joined him in the bedroom to get myself ready. He was leaning against the bed, hunkered over struggling with the buttons on the sleeve of his dress shirt.

We have an agreement that I won't offer help unless he asks. I was dressed and ready to go, but Mike was still working on the second sleeve.

"Damn!" he muttered from across the room.

I found some clothes to fold at the end of the bed. After a few minutes, Mike advanced to the row of shirt buttons. He always starts with the second to the bottom button, and works his way to the top, leaving the bottom button undone.

Pretty soon, I heard another louder expression of frustration. Luckily, I had sheets to fold. Finally, Mike let loose with the defining profanity, so I went across the room to help him button his shirt. He looked completely worn out, and the evening was only beginning.

When I finished the buttoning, he said, "Thanks for the help." Then he made one of his amusing and endearing observations: "Buttoning my shirt is like trying to build a Model T with a sled."

After living with Parkinson's for so long, I have learned that Mike can do only one thing at a time. To succeed at anything, he must focus on one task until it is finished. When presented with simultaneous tasks—emotional, physical, or mental—his ability to complete any single task to his satisfaction dwindles into frustration.

One Thing At a Time

People with Parkinson's do not need to apologize. Their limitations do not mean they have done something wrong. It's simply a matter of educating patients, caregivers, families, and the general public.

Macy's Department Store, Bellingham, Washington:

Excuse me, young man? Could you help me? I need a black suit. Size 38.

What is the occasion, sir?

I'm going to the White House

Did you say the White House, Sir?

Yes, the Correspondent's Christmas Party. My son invited me. I have a message for the President.

We'll have to tailor these pants, Sir.

I must be shrinking.

Excuse me, sir? Did you say sinking?

I'm sorry, I have Parkinson's disease. Sometimes it's hard to understand me. I said shrinking.

Oh, yes. I'm sorry, sir. My grandfather has Parkinson's, too. He used to be a farmer.

I used to be an artist. I'd like that Garcia tie. And a coral, silk . . . short-sleeved dress shirt.

9:00 A.M. Pacific Standard Time, Northwest Terminal Sea-Tac Airport, 3,478 miles to go:

Himself. His hand-carved maple cane with the cherry wood handle. His very own Parkinson's disease. And his message.

4:00 P.M. Eastern Standard Time, Washington D.C.

Belt looped in black suit pants—6 minutes. Eight small buttons on coral silk shirt—4 minutes per button. Garcia tie knotted—12 minutes. Walk through the door—2 minutes. Message in pocket.

5:30 P.M. Official limousine arrives.

Bulletproof windows, snow on the road, slippery, *could be late, can't be late. Don't look outside. Don't talk to the driver. Just focus on the message.*

6:00 P.M. arrival at the White House.

Under the portico, red carpet. Secret Service, CIA buffed in black leather. The West Wing. *Awesome power. Concentrate on the door, the door.* Christmas lights, music, surveillance, clearance, speed.

Name, Sir? Social Security number, Sir? Guest of? You are a guest of whom? Sir? All right. Cleared! Right through that door. Follow that escort.

Another door. He freezes in the doorway, stutters forward, almost falling. Recovers.

Sir? Line up here and keep moving. You'll have 10 seconds. Shake the President's hand. Have your picture taken. It's important to keep moving.

Ten, nine, eight, seven. Half a handshake away. Inside his black suit, cell phone rings. *Too many deep pockets.* Fumbling, stumbling, feet stuttering, arms flailing. Cane flies, message aloft. Secret Service advances. Bush's hand appears, official camera flashes.

Sir! Keep moving . . . . Sir. He freezes but his carefully written 5-second message keeps moving. Stuck to the ribbed heel of the secret service agent. *Please, Mr. President, reconsider your policy on stem cell research.*

Stem cells are cells found in most, if not all, multicellular organisms. They are characterized by the ability to renew themselves through mitotic cell division and have the capacity to differentiate into a diverse range of specialized cell types. Stem cells hold the possibility for treatments and cures for many ailments, including Parkinson's disease.

President George W. Bush limited funding for stem cell research, and in May 2005, he vowed to veto a compromise (that would have repealed the 2001 limits on spending) that 50 Republicans and 188 Democrats in the House of Representatives supported. In March of 2009, President Obama lifted the Bush administration's strict limits on human stem cell research, thus increasing the possibilities for fruitful research in this important area of science.

After his experience at the White House, Mike carries a plastic I.D. tag with him for security when he goes to unfamiliar places. In bold letters it reads: *I'm sorry, I have Parkinson's disease. Sometimes it's hard for me to walk and talk.*

Imagine someone apologizing for an illness. Imponderable as it is, that's just what Mike does. Invariably, after a couple of failed attempts to explain something to a stranger, Mike begins again by saying, "I'm sorry, I have Parkinson's disease." Then he has the person's attention. He apologizes for the obvious inconvenience his condition presents to others.

One afternoon, Mike entered a hardware store in downtown Bellingham, but he froze in the open doorway. A man in a wheelchair rolled up to him.

"Boy, I know how it feels to get stuck in a door," the man said. "Let me give you a hand." Such compassion: The paraplegic in a wheelchair offering a hand to the person with PD stuck in a doorway.

Again, Mike said, "I'm sorry, I have Parkinson's disease. It always takes me a few minutes to get through a doorway."

Inside the Parkinson's Community

According to the practice of "direct contact," if we wish to understand any culture we must live within that community—not just observe and analyze others from the outside. We must have meaningful contact with each other, including our health care providers.

The practice of "direct contact" is something we once took for granted, especially in our doctor–patient relationships. This is no longer the case.

At the First World Parkinson's Congress, held in Washington D.C. in 2006, Mike and I were among 1,000 people with Parkinson's disease (PD) and their caregivers, as we joined an international group of doctors and researchers converging on the D.C. convention center. On the second day of breakout sessions, over 200 people with PD and caregivers eagerly crowded into a presentation room to hear a doctor with PD and his caregiver wife tell their personal story.

The atmosphere in the room was palpably restless. Almost before the speakers were finished, hands were flying in the air. These people had anxious questions. Caregivers were desperate for answers. "Who do I call?" asked an admittedly worn-out elderly sister and caregiver of a man in the back of the room. "We live in the country," she cried, "I can't leave him alone. We don't have a support network."

Many of the caregivers were frantic for information, guidance, and support. As the questions fired off from dozens of concerned people, I noticed a woman my daughter's age sitting next to me. She was crying. She was too young for this. I reached over to touch her arm, and her body shook as she told me that her husband was just diagnosed.

"He's only 40 years old," she whispered, with tears flowing down her face. "We have little kids. I don't know what to do or what to expect. It's really scary and he's really angry. He totally does not believe it."

All I could do was look back at her and attempt to convey understanding and compassion.

The second speaker was a physician, a Parkinson's specialist. First, he thanked us for the opportunity to observe so many patients and caregivers in community.

"As physicians," the doctor began with a tone of regret, "we don't have the luxury of listening to you for more than 15 minutes per appointment—just a few times a year. Being with you in this atmosphere here at the conference is a rare gift. I have seen how you work together in community. I've observed how the more functional patients step forward to help the less able through doorways, on and off the escalators, and in the dining room. I can see that caregivers do everything possible to make patients feel normal and comfortable."

Those of us who care for people with PD do indeed *live* in what often appears to be an incomprehensible situation. It is up to us to employ and promote successful strategies in the care of persons with Parkinson's, and in the care of ourselves, especially in complex situations.

For example, something as simple as planning an evening "out" can become complicated, because Mike should eat within half an hour of taking his Sinemet®. Without the medication, his body becomes rigid and he is unable to move. If he eats earlier than half an hour after taking his medication, its benefits are drastically reduced. If he waits too long, he becomes agitated, has more difficulty talking, chewing, and swallowing, and also runs the risk of biting his tongue from chewing too fast.

When we entertain at home, Mike has to first make a decision. If he wants to visit with guests, he does not take his medication; if he wants to have the flexibility to get up from the table, he takes his medication—but he cannot both visit and walk.

With this delicate balance in mind, on a lovely spring evening we were invited to attend readings presented by graduate students in the English department at Western Washington University. The program was scheduled to begin at 7:00 P.M. and would last about an hour and a half.

At 5:30, Mike took his medication and we went downtown for dinner. The restaurant was packed, the service was slow, and Mike couldn't chew much of what he ordered because it was too long after his meds. To make matters worse, I misunderstood the time and precise location of the readings. It started at 7:30 and was on the second floor, 30-plus steps from street level. The program lasted longer than anticipated, continuing for over 2 hours, by which time Mike could feel his medication wearing off. In a few unpredictable moments, he would be rigid and barely able to walk back down the stairs.

We managed to stay till the end of the program, and then we made a clumsy and ungracious departure through the back door, only to discover it was pouring rain. Halfway down the stairs, and gripping my arm for dear life, Mike said, "Make a break for the street and get to the car as fast as you can, before I turn into a pumpkin."

Mike and I have created a bridge, a new language, to facilitate our conversations. Because he sometimes has trouble enunciating, I have difficulty understanding what he's saying. To complicate matters Mike has a hearing deficit, caused by a childhood accident, and he does not always hear what I'm saying. So, I repeat what I think he said and he repeats what he thinks he heard me say. The result is usually much more entertaining and satisfying than our original statements. For instance on our anniversary last year we had dinner at a restaurant overlooking the North Sound. It was buzzing with conversation, glasses tinkling, waiters delivering detailed descriptions of seasonal local oysters and too-distracting yummy combinations of vegetables and salmon, halibut, and squash with fruit demi-glaces.

Through the cacophony I asked Mike a question, which now I don't even recall.

"Pardon?" he asked, cupping his good ear. I repeated the question. Again he said, "Pardon me?"

I grabbed a pen and leaned across the white tablecloth. I spoke as clearly as I could without raising my voice for everyone in the restaurant to hear.

"Pretty soon," I warned him, "I will start writing on the table."

He looked startled and said, "You'll do *what* with Clark Gable?"

Bronislaw Malinowski (1884–1942), known as the Father of Social Anthropology, might refer to this kind of language adaptation as *phatic communion*. We are at one with each other. We are communicating and bonding using the tools available to us at the moment.

Malinowski believed in bringing anthropology *off the verandah*, meaning that researchers must have daily contact with their subjects—integrating details and synthesizing various relevant symptoms—if they are to accurately record and respond to what he referred to as *the imponderabilia of everyday life*.

Art As a Lifeline

I am an artist in my mind and in my soul. There is something I can still do.

Mike dictated the following artist's statement in response to a request for proposals for an art exhibit to be displayed at the World Parkinson's Congress in 2006:

"Art has been my passion since 1956, when I was a graduate student and discovered my first mentor, Frances Senska, in the ceramics department at Montana State University in Bozeman. She gave me 'legs.'

"After more than 30 years of making pots, Parkinson's disease gained ground in my muscles, and I had to explore less physically demanding methods of pursuing my art. After 7 years of welding huge metal sculptures, I could no longer lift or move heavy objects.

"Sometimes, I could not move myself or safely walk to or around my studio without the fear of freezing and falling. I sat on a stool and looked out the window, wondering, 'What can I do now?'

"Today, the strength in my legs is more limited, but I am still an artist—in my mind and in my soul. That is exactly what I have left, and I will use my mind the best way I am able."

The popular singer, Chris Isaak, sings of the yellow bird. Mike relates to the lyrics, longing to be like the yellow bird, graceful and free. He's discouraged and worries that there is nothing left for him to do. He sits in his studio, fearful that he may end up doing nothing more with his life than sitting.

"Big, bold, colossal statements have been replaced in my life with the simplicity and power of symbols. For me, it has become more critical to convey essence and meaning.

"My yellow seagull [sculpture] symbolizes the freedom that eludes people with Parkinson's disease. There is an adjustable nut on the back of the yellow bird that allows for dependable and graceful movement. The color yellow symbolizes hope, courage, and perseverance, all of which have been critical for me in recognizing and embracing the continuing and exciting possibilities for the creation of art in my life.

"I am the orange gull—different from the others, but still standing—and there *is* something I can still do."

Mike's yellow seagull sculptures may be viewed at
www.yellowbirdsforparkinsons.com.

When a Spouse Becomes a Caregiver*

Nanette J. Davis, Ph.D.

A nne and Mike Mikkelsen demonstrate that it is possible to live well, and even thrive, despite the problems that Parkinson's disease (PD) brings to their relationship. In their willingness to both give and receive for one another, each has also discovered the remarkable and life-sustaining gifts of care partnering. Their story shows us that caregiving need not be characterized only by fear and anxiety—the experience can ultimately be freeing and joyful.

THE CHALLENGES OF CARE PARTNERING

Much has been written about the "burden" of care: the 24/7 day, the "reluctant caregiver" and other, less positive, aspects of the caregiving experience such as a lack of access to support and resources, and the issue of "caregiver burnout." This "no-relief-in-sight" formula undermines both carepartners.

Instead, caregiving can be regarded as a strategy that focuses on the benefits and rewards of being in *partnership*, even while living with a serious disease. Focusing on the positive aspects of caregiving allows us the freedom to pursue our lives, while at the same time following our partner's progress.

---

*More reflections on caregiving can be found in *Blessed Is She: Women's Stories of Choice, Challenge and Commitment* by Nanette J. David, Ph.D.

The challenges of caregiving can reshape our concept of giving as we recognize what our carepartner is still able to do, rather than dwelling on the limitations imposed by PD. This will allow you to become open to a deeper level of awareness in day-to-day life.

NINE POSITIVE ASPECTS OF CARE PARTNERING

There are nine "gifts" that can be brought to the care partnership as a result of a creative and open perspective:

1. *Having an open heart.* Wisdom of the heart brings intuition and love into every aspect of the caregiving relationship. Act on the certain recognition of the circle of life: You will both give *and* receive along your journey. Keeping this in mind can help you gradually shift from seeing caregiving only as a duty and responsibility to more positive thinking— taking the high road.

2. *Connecting with the generations.* Anne cultivates her relationships with sisters, adult children, and grandchildren, as well as with Mike's family members. Everyone who cares to participate is part of the fabric of kinship. Family stories, traditions, and activities—especially cooking— structure their days and provide a wealth of meaning for everyone. Even neighbors and friends are brought into the fold—some to help Mike, others to help sustain Anne's energies during difficult times.

3. *Expanding your coping abilities.* When a family or partnership crisis happens, it is tempting to simply allow things to fall apart and to forego the opportunity to expand your coping abilities. Anne has developed more effective and life-renewing strategies. Through the years, she has learned to accept *what is*, rather than strive for *what can never be* or *what should be*. A successful business owner and community organizer, she turned her creative skills into domestic accomplishments, mastering the art of cooking nutritious and delicious food that may slow down the progress

of PD. Developing new routines helps both carepartners, as they make a concerted effort to appreciate each other's needs and aspirations.

Like most successful caregivers, Anne has developed management skills that go beyond her entrepreneurial and culinary endeavors. She has learned to effectively deal with the often resistant health care system and to coordinate an effective care program for her husband. In many cases, this requires a somewhat confrontational manner. After all, the "soft" voice is often overlooked in today's medical and bureaucratic worlds.

4. *Willingness to experience role reversal.* Perhaps one of the more difficult tests caregivers face is the inevitable role reversal that occurs when one partner must cope with a growing inability to perform what previously had been their "normal" roles. A wife may need to take on tasks such as mowing the yard, a task formerly done by her husband, or a husband may have to take on unfamiliar chores such as cooking. An abrupt stand of "taking over" a task does not work. Rather, a heartfelt willingness to do whatever must be done to maintain sanity and well-being for both partners will save the day

5. *Reinvigorating family relationships.* Ideally, caregiving brings all family members together to achieve a common goal: giving comfort and aid to the person with PD, as well as respite for the primary caregiver. This may not always be possible if ties have been broken and a spirit of collaboration no longer exists. Both carepartners should make a concerted effort to get all family members to put aside their individual differences and develop a sense of team work. This will benefit everyone.

6. *Strengthening bonds with the community.* Reaching out to your community can lead to making new friendships and allies. Anne serves as an advocate for Mike, a role that involves working with the national and regional PD community, as well as his medical providers. Advocating for our partners involves speaking up when they cannot. This gives us a sense of purpose and accomplishment, and shows them how deeply we care.

7. *Giving back to others.* The act of putting another person before oneself is an essential part of maintaining the fabric of our society. Think of

parents, rescue teams, firefighters, and others whose job is to put the needs of others before their own. Psychologists tell us that bringing help and joy to others is a "feel-good" experience, and becomes its own reward: in giving, we receive.

8. *Expressing our spiritual values.* The challenges of providing long-term care are enormous, and watching a loved one deteriorate can be especially difficult. For PD carepartners, the road can be so very long—what seems like a lifetime. We have to reach inside for our very survival. Caregiving becomes a transforming experience when we act on our core beliefs: faith in the future, hope, and love.

9. *The importance of self-care.* Taking care of your physical, mental, and emotional health is a top priority for every caregiver. No matter how much you try to be positive about the caregiving experience, you still must maintain a sense of yourself and be aware of your own needs. Otherwise, you will lose your sense of self, which can result in your own health problems, both physical and emotional. To avoid this, it is essential that you develop clear personal boundaries, and carve out time for yourself each and every day. This may require accepting your own limitations and asking for help. Anne's strategy has been to remind herself that no one person can do it all.

REDUCING CAREGIVER STRESS

Here are a few suggestions that can help you reduce daily stress and help sustain you as a caregiver:

▶ Start a regular exercise program that is realistic for your lifestyle and age.
▶ Strengthen your social network within your own community.
▶ Work at following a well-balanced diet, one that emphasizes fruit, vegetables, and grains.
▶ Avoid excessive eating or drinking.

▶ Breathe deeply throughout the day.
▶ Quiet the mind with meditation, yoga, reading, prayer, or other practices.
▶ Be impassioned about your life.

Changing the Culinary Repertoire

The key to success in living with Parkinson's disease is implementing an entire lifestyle approach that includes good nutrition, exercise, stress management, and using the lowest effective doses of medications.

During a Parkinson's conference in 2005, I listened with interest to the rationale for a diet low in animal protein and rich in antioxidants and nutrient-dense plant foods. My first thought was, "He's talking about hippy food that looks and tastes like cardboard."

However, the presentation seemed credible enough, because the speaker was a physician who also had Parkinson's disease (PD). He outlined a compelling case for a lifestyle that just might make a difference, including eating certain foods as a possible means of slowing the progression of Parkinson's.

On the stage beside the speaker, there was an overhead photograph of foods that contain high levels of antioxidants, but he made it clear that simply eating a bowl of blueberries every week, or even every day, was not the total answer. He suggested that the key to success is an entire lifestyle that includes good nutrition, exercise, stress management, and using the lowest effective doses of medications.

Good nutrition means eating less animal-based food and adding the widest variety of nutrient-dense, naturally low-calorie foods, such as fresh fruits and vegetables, whole grains, and occasionally animal-based foods such as salmon, free-range chickens, and eggs.

My response was spontaneous: we needed to add more plant-based ingredients to our diet. Mike and I had already established a regular exercise routine—and because of Mike's stubbornness, he was already taking the lowest dose of medication. However, we also needed to eliminate some foods, because our diet was top-heavy with dairy and meat. Our table partners at the conference were equally inspired, but expressed realistic reservations. "How the heck would you combine those ingredients and make them taste good?"

I had doubts about my ability to give up my dependence on so many familiar and comforting ingredients—foods I'd literally cut my culinary teeth on. I saw a great portion of my repertoire flying out the kitchen windows, leaving garlic, lemons, and my pepper grinder standing alone on the chopping block. Fortunately, I would soon learn this image was delusional.

The sustaining and empowering take-away message from the convention was that people with PD and caregivers *can do* something; they can take action every day, three times a day or more, to positively affect the quality of their lives.

T. Colin Campbell makes a beautiful point in his book *The China Study: Startling Implications for Diet, Weight Loss and Long-Term Health* about the synergism of just one single plant. His words give me courage:

> The triumph of health lies not in the individual nutrients, but in the whole foods that contain those nutrients: plant-based foods. In a bowl of spinach, for example, we have fiber, antioxidants, and countless other nutrients that are orchestrating a wondrous symphony of health as they work in concert within our bodies.

One of our primary purposes in writing this book is to spread the excitement and array of our low-fat, brain-healthy pantry. In Part II, we will introduce you to some possibilities for delicious savory meals loaded with antioxidants and anti-inflammatory substances known to benefit brain health. Through our story and recipes, we hope to inspire you to create your own recipes using the dynamic list of healthy ingredients.

PART II

Food and Optimal Wellness
with Parkinson's Disease

What Are Free Radicals and Antioxidants?

Free radicals are unstable atoms that contain unpaired electrons. They are formed during a process called *oxidation*, and are produced naturally in the body. They can also be produced in excess by environmental conditions such as pollution, ultraviolet rays, cigarette smoking, and radiation. They damage cells throughout the body because they "steal" electrons from other cells in order to become "complete" through electron pairing. This results in even more instability and more damage to cells. In turn, an ongoing chain reaction of cell damage is triggered that, over time, can increase the risk of many types of disease, as well as speed up the aging process.

Unchecked free radical activity has been linked to Parkinson's disease (PD), in large part because the neurons that use dopamine as their neurotransmitter are especially vulnerable to injury caused by oxidation—and as already discussed, low levels of dopamine are known to contribute to the development of PD.

Antioxidants can stop the free radical chain reaction, thereby protecting cells from further oxidative damage. Antioxidants include vitamins, minerals, and other nutrients found in many foods, such as vegetables, fruits, grain cereals, eggs, meat, legumes, nuts, and certain culinary herbs and spices. The three major antioxidant vitamins are beta-carotene, vitamin C, and vitamin E. These are found primarily in colorful fruits and vegetables, especially those with purple, blue, red, orange, and yellow hues. Processed foods generally contain fewer antioxidants than fresh and uncooked foods. Dried fruits are also a good source.

Black and green teas, and certain herbs such as thyme, are very rich sources of a specific kind of antioxidant called *flavonoids*, chemical compounds produced by plants to protect their cells from damage. Evidence suggests that flavonoids may play a role in reversing the loss of neurons in neurodegenerative disease.

It's All About Lifestyle

A healthy lifestyle requires flexibility and a willingness to adapt—sometimes on short notice!

Mike once responded to someone who correctly observed that I own an *un-fussy* assortment of cooking implements. "If she has the ingredients she wants," he said, "she'll cook it in a shoe if she has to."

My favorite pans are cast iron, and I have five in three sizes. I also own a crepe pan and a copper stockpot that I bought in France—and I admit that we built both our Northfield and Bellingham kitchens around professional, six-burner gas stoves.

Every meal is an event, beginning the moment you first imagine the smell and taste of an herb combined with a particular fresh raw ingredient. The event only ends when the memory of what you created is replaced by the inspiration for another meal.

For instance, imagine the tantalizing aroma of rosemary gently toasting in extra virgin olive oil, or the fragrance of garlic sautéing with sweet red peppers, onions, parsley, thyme, and the effervescence of sweet knotted marjoram. These ingredients are just the beginning, the base for an antioxidant-rich hearty soup.

The recipes in the next section are primarily plant-based. They are not fast food, nor are they complicated. They are designed specifically for home cooks, which is exactly how I was first introduced to the magic of cooking by my Grandma White.

Home cooking has always sustained Mike and me. In Bellingham, where it seems that every household has at least one garden, I frequently hear people say, "You are what you plant." I believe this is true, and so it follows that *we are what we eat*, and *each body sings its own symphony*.

Even if you don't have access to fruits and vegetables from your own garden, good, fresh ingredients are available almost everywhere.

I returned home to the kitchen from the Parkinson's conference with renewed enthusiasm and an inspiring list of neuroprotective antioxidants added to the already expansive pantry we've enjoyed for years.

Moderation is considered wise in most endeavors, but with PD present in our lives we choose to combine the *widest variety of antioxidant ingredients*— and we try to avoid foods that might exacerbate the symptoms of PD.

As the doctor said, "There is no single 'magic bullet.'" Our formula is really about a *lifestyle*. It is not perfect, and it will not reverse the ravages of Parkinson's disease, but we strive for a do-no-harm approach. If this seems idealistic, it is! I know Mike thinks about his PD symptoms every day, but he proudly acknowledges the importance of daily exercise and healthy eating:

"Every day is like walking over ice on a snowy road. At all times, I have to be observant of the space in front of me. Be aware of any unevenness—on the road I walk, the hours I sleep, the meds I take, the food I eat. I may not like that fact, but I do accept it. I'm forced to assess my symptoms every day for my own safety. . .and my remaining independence.

"Getting out of bed each morning, I begin by surveying my surroundings. Now, I'm getting closer to falling every time I get up—even from my chair. Am I on solid footing today? Is my cane beside me? If not, can I move without my cane? Next, where is it? I calculate how I can get my body to another place by locating furniture to hang on to, careful to anticipate the distance I can safely traverse. There's always that walker lurking down in the basement. I do not want to fall, I know the consequences. This is my valley. But every barrier is a springboard for a new direction of thought. I'd like to see an electronic device, laptop, with the capability of reading my brain waves, sensing my thoughts. By the touch of my finger this device could communicate my feelings in words like a normal conversation.

"Every day I realize that time is closing in. I used to think, *Oh, they'll find a cure, then this monkey will be off my back and I will go forward.* But now advancing age has come into play and something will take me out. I can't avoid that, so I accept it and appreciate the everyday gifts in front of me—the smile on my wife's face is like an injection of serotonin that makes looking at my life a positive reflection. I'm proud that I haven't let PD completely take over my life. In addition, I have a lifestyle that allows me to pursue what I love: living in the country, still getting my own firewood, and creating my art."

While we're at it, let's not forget the importance of *how* we eat, which may be almost as important as *what* we eat. How often do we find ourselves sitting at a table, or instead standing beside the microwave, running out the door with a packaged meal, or driving through a fast-food lane? Are we relaxed and enjoying the experience of eating? Our style of eating may have a lot to do with our level of stress—and vice-versa.

The Brain-Healthy Pantry

My personal list of "wonder ingredients" includes salmon, extra virgin olive oil, lemons, limes, garlic, black pepper, red peppers, tomatoes, eggplant, squash, blueberries, blackberries, walnuts, pine nuts, hazelnuts, ginger root, sweet onions, and dried sour cherries. These ingredients and those that follow represent versatility and dependability. They can be inspiring in the quest to prepare healthy food.

ANTIOXIDANT-RICH SPICES AND HERBS

When possible, try to use the *widest* variety of fresh herbs: rosemary, basil, parsley, marjoram, dill, French tarragon, oregano, cilantro, thyme, lovage, sage, mint, and sorrel. By all means, use dried herbs when fresh are not available. The general rule for fresh to dried herb conversion is 1 tsp dried to 1 T fresh, but use your judgment and season to taste.

Here are some other good items to have on hand:

- *Spices and seeds.* Turmeric, nutmeg, cinnamon, cloves, ginger, coriander (seeds of cilantro), caraway seed, poppy seed, a variety of red pepper spices, cumin, dill seeds, and regular white and black sesame seeds
- *Grains.* Sweet brown rice, Israeli couscous, barley, flax seed, wild rice, quinoa, and soba noodles
- *Dried beans.* Black beans, pinto beans, black-eyed peas, lentils, fava beans, and cannellini beans

▶ *Nuts.* Walnuts, pecans, pine nuts, almonds, hazelnuts, sunflower seeds, and pumpkin seeds

Certain culinary spices and herbs are considered a more concentrated source of dietary antioxidants than many other food groups:

▶ Cinnamon has one of the highest antioxidant levels of any spice. One teaspoon of cinnamon contains as many antioxidants as a full cup of pomegranate juice or a half-cup of blueberries.

▶ *Carnosic acid*, a component in rosemary, increases the body's production of glutathione, one of the most important antioxidants that may help protect the brain against free radical damage.

▶ Oregano has one of the highest antioxidant levels of all dried herbs. One teaspoon of dried oregano leaves has as many antioxidants as 3 ounces of almonds or a half-cup of chopped asparagus.

▶ A teaspoon of thyme contains about the same amount of antioxidants as a carrot or a half-cup of chopped tomatoes. Thyme also contains a variety of flavonoids that increase its antioxidant capacity and may offer anti-inflammatory benefits.

▶ Turmeric, found in curry powder, is a concentrated source of antioxidants—on a par with strawberries, raspberries, and cherries. One teaspoon of curry powder has as many antioxidants as a half-cup of red grapes. Emerging evidence suggests that curcumin, which gives turmeric its bright yellow color, may reduce inflammation and help safeguard the brain.

Gadgets You'll Never Regret Owning

Tools that I use regularly that you might consider: vegetable steamer, pasta machine, lettuce spinner, lemon zester, nutmeg grater, and a good pepper grinder.

▶ Cayenne pepper is a potent antioxidant. Along with other "red pepper" spices, including chili powder and paprika, cayenne also contains *capsaicin*, which inhibits the inflammatory process.

FOOD TOOLS TO KEEP STOCKED IN YOUR PANTRY

The "food tools" described here are used in many of the recipes in this collection. In addition to possessing multiple antioxidant ingredients, each has its own function and allure, either as a foundation or an accessory.

Olive Oil

In all of the recipes below, "olive oil" means *extra virgin* olive oil. We also use canola oil, which has significant amounts of the desirable inflammatory-reducing omega-3 fatty acids.

Lemons and Limes

We use a lot of lemons and limes in our recipes—at least six lemons a week and even more limes if I'm using the smaller Key lime variety. I've always included these fresh, lively flavors because they add vibrancy and pizzazz to every ingredient they touch. Since we moved to Bellingham—where many of the grocers display lemons in huge wire baskets—I have adopted them as a necessary staple. Plus, using more lemon juice means you can use less salt.

In addition to tasting good, lemons and limes contain unique flavonoid compounds and are an excellent source of vitamin C, one of the most important antioxidants found in nature.

The two main types of sour lemons are the Eureka and the Lisbon. The Eureka has a more textured skin, a short neck at one end, and a few seeds. The Lisbon has a smoother skin, no neck, and is mostly seedless.

Ah, but there is another lemon with all the healing properties of the sour lemons and additional qualities if you are looking for a more subtle flavor. The

Meyer lemon—a cross between the common lemon and the mandarin orange—is smoother, sweeter, sometimes darker in color, and totally eatable, including the skin. Meyer lemons work deliciously with all ingredients, especially delicate fish preparations, salads, and desserts. So you have three options for lemons: Meyer, Eureka, and Lisbon.

The most common lime is the true lime, which is larger than the Key limes that are thin-skinned and have an intense tropical flavor. The Mexican sweet lime, also thin-skinned, has a sweeter flavor and is nearly without acidity.

You will soon notice that I use a lot of fresh lemons and lemon zest. If juice and zest are both called for in a recipe, I suggest you remove the zest first, then slice and juice the lemon.

Teas and Coffee

We use three different teas every day: Earl Grey in the morning before breakfast, Genmaicha green tea for lunch, and blueberry Rooibos in the afternoon.

Mike has trouble sleeping at night, so we went on a hunt for a good caffeine-free tea, and we discovered we like the red and blueberry Rooibos teas. Among its other attributes, the Rooibos teas are extremely high in antioxidants.

Genmaicha is Japanese green leaf tea combined with ground-roasted rice. It smells rich and comforting while brewing. The rice gives it a distinctive nutty, roasted flavor. Genmaicha is high in antioxidants, including tannins and flavonoids, which are powerful companions when combined with lemon.

Earl Grey is a black tea also known for its antioxidant properties.

We only drink coffee in the morning with breakfast.

Pepper

Fresh ground black pepper stimulates the taste buds, which is very important because diminishing taste is a common feature of Parkinson's disease (and aging), and we need all the help we can get! Pepper also helps promote digestion. Grinding pepper exclusively at the moment you need it helps preserve the flavor.

Pepper is also a good activator of herbs; for example, pepper added to turmeric increases the potency of the turmeric.

Sea Salts

If you want to add salt to your food, try using sea salt. Because of its more intense flavor, people tend to use less of it. There are so many exciting flavors, from chipotle to lemon, merlot, and lavender. I love the smoky sea salt for its versatility. You could even try making your own blend by combining plain sea salt with fresh or dried herbs, or you can make a rub by combining sea salt with herbs and pepper in a coffee grinder. Whirl the mixture until well blended and rub onto fish or chicken before cooking, or sprinkle it lightly on steamed vegetables.

Cucumbers

There's nothing wrong with the common slicing cucumber, but the English cucumber—if available—has it beat in several ways:

- ▶ English cucumbers are generally sold wrapped in plastic to reduce water loss, and so they are usually not waxed and therefore do not need peeling.
- ▶ They usually called "seedless" (which is not true), but the seeds *are* much smaller and less prominent.
- ▶ The seeds in cucumbers (especially in aging cucumbers) make them bitter, so a semi-seedless English cucumber is less likely to be bitter.
- ▶ English cucumbers have been bred to be more easily digested than some other varieties (read: fewer burps).

Onions

Onions are yellow, white, or red, with yellow being the most common. They are low in saturated fat, cholesterol, and sodium. Onions are a good source of dietary fiber, vitamin B$_6$, potassium, manganese, and an excellent source of vitamin C.

There are two basic categories of onions, spring/summer and fall/winter. The spring/summer onions are known as "fresh market" onions. They have a thinner, paler skin, and they are mostly sweeter and less pungent than fall/winter onions.

Fall/winter onions have thicker skin, more layers, a stronger flavor, a longer storage life, and less variety than spring/summer onions. Fall/winter onions are the most common type available.

One of the larger varieties of sweet onion is the Walla Walla Sweet, grown in Walla Walla, Washington. They are available in many states from June to August. Because this prized onion tastes so good and is grown in Washington, I like to use it whenever I can. Sweet onions don't cause tears when you chop them and they caramelize beautifully when sautéed, adding just the right amount of sweetness to any preparation.

Other American sweet onions that might be available in your area include: the super sweet onions grown in Texas, available March through August; Vidalia onions from Georgia, available nationwide April through June; Grand Canyon Sweets grown in Arizona, available May to June; Maui Sweet Onions from Hawaii, available year-round; Nu Mex Sweet from New Mexico, available June through August; and Sweet Imperials from Southern California, the most widely produced sweet onion, available from April to September. When sweet onions are not available, use fall/winter onions—but use onions!

PANTRY PREPARATION TECHNIQUES

To peel fresh tomatoes: Place tomatoes in a large bowl. Boil enough water to cover them. When water is boiling, pour over tomatoes (do not boil tomatoes).

Let stand in boiling water 1–3 minutes, or until skin becomes loose. Pour off water and peel tomatoes.

To roast a red pepper: Roast a sweet red pepper on a grill or on top of the stove with the burner set on high. Turn pepper until entire coat is blackened. Place charred pepper in a bowl to cool. Peel all the charred skin off. *Do not wash* the pepper. Use paper towel to wipe off extra charred bits. Discard the seeds and slice or chop the pepper.

A note about garlic: If you want the health benefits of garlic, but not the strong odor, try this trick. Drop a clove of unpeeled garlic into boiling water and leave it for a minute. Remove garlic, peel and mash. Whisk into your recipe.

Roasted Rosemary

There is new research on loss of smell as an early predictor of PD. Mike remembers losing his sense of smell long before his first PD symptoms appeared. He can still taste some random ingredients, especially potatoes, and he can always taste the first bite of anything. Some ingredients trigger his olfactory receptors more than others. He always expresses a positive response to the aroma of roasting rosemary. "I've always loved fruit, the textures, the sweetness, but I can catch the zest of those herbs every once in a while, and that's a treat."

Roasting rosemary provides more possibilities for use of this beneficial herb, especially because fresh rosemary can be difficult for people with PD to chew. Because of its dominant taste, the uses for rosemary are somewhat limited to robust meat preparations; but once roasted, the herb is crunchy and easier to chew, and the flavor is subtler. Roasted rosemary is more sociable when combined with delicate ingredients.

An added benefit of roasting rosemary is the heart-warming, exhilarating aroma that will fill your home. It feels like someone loves you, even if you're the one doing the roasting!

To roast rosemary, preheat oven to 350 degrees. Place rosemary branches on a baking sheet and sprinkle with a little canola oil. Bake for 12–15 minutes, or

Rosemary has been shown to improve circulation and stimulate the brain, so it is frequently described as *the herb of memory*. Rosemary is a well-established anti-inflammatory.

Rosmarinic acid, an important constituent of rosemary, has powerful antioxidant and preservative qualities.

Rosemary gets its name from the Latin words meaning: "dew" and "of the sea." Rosemary is a piney-scented herb that makes us, and our taste buds, happy. Try to incorporate rosemary in as many dishes as possible. To make this plant even more versatile, included below is a recipe for oven-toasting rosemary.

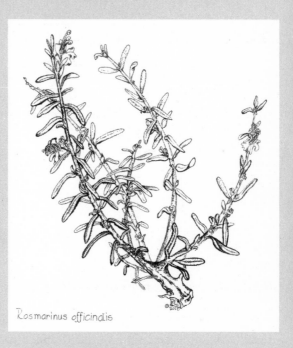

Rosmarinus officinalis

until the color has changed to khaki green but not brown. Every oven is a little different, so watch the rosemary closely the first time you try this. If you roast it to dark brown, the taste will range from bitter to nothing. Remove from baking sheet and drain on paper towel. At this stage, the leaves are ready to use, but if you want to save the roasted rosemary, wait until it is totally cooled, wrap it in a fresh paper towel, and store it in an air-tight container for up to a week. Roasted rosemary is good sprinkled on cooked pizza, meats, fish, and vegetables.

REFRIGERATED PANTRY PREPARATIONS

The next eight preparations are loaded with antioxidants, and they will contribute excitement to almost anything you serve. We refer to these multipurpose essentials as *rescuers*, because they add another unexpected dimension of visual and taste sensation to any dish.

Tomato Base

¼ cup extra virgin olive oil

½ cup onion, chopped

5 large, ripe, peeled tomatoes, chopped (or two 14-ounce cans of stewed tomatoes with oregano and basil)

3 cloves garlic, minced

½ cup fresh basil

2 T oregano

1 T sweet marjoram

1 tsp turmeric

1½ cup water

1 tsp salt and 2 grinds of cracked pepper

Heat 3 T olive oil in a medium-sized saucepan. Add onions and stir over medium heat until caramelized. Add chopped tomatoes (or canned stewed tomatoes) garlic, basil, oregano, marjoram, turmeric, and water. Cook sauce over medium heat, stirring until slightly thickened. Add remaining tablespoon of olive oil, salt and pepper. You can store this base, tightly covered, in the refrigerator for a week. Makes approximately 4 cups of red sauce.

Black Olive Tower

We call this "the new gravy" because, among other uses, it works well as a topping for mashed potatoes, replacing the traditional gravy recipes that were loaded with butter and cream.

2 T red wine vinegar

4 T olive oil

½ tsp salt and cracked pepper

1 cucumber diced (I prefer English cucumbers; pound for pound they are more economical because you can use the entire fruit—skin, seeds, and all)

3 medium tomatoes, peeled

½ cup onion, chopped

½ cup black Kalamata olives, chopped (to me, Kalamata olives have a better texture and taste)

2 cloves garlic, chopped

½ avocado, chopped

1 T fresh basil or cilantro, chopped

Combine oil and vinegar with salt and pepper. Add cucumber, tomatoes, onions, olives, garlic, and avocado. Stir. Just before using, add fresh chopped herbs and mix again. Makes 2 cups.

Lemon/Onion/Caper/Walnut Relish

Zest of one whole lemon (set aside)

Juice of 1 whole lemon about 1 T

1 T olive oil

½ medium sweet onion, sliced and rings separated

½ cup toasted and slightly crushed black walnuts

1 T capers

Place onion rings into bowl and squeeze lemon juice over. Add olive oil and marinate for 1 hour. Toast walnuts on a baking sheet in 350 degree oven until they smell done, about 12 minutes. Crush walnuts over onion rings and add capers. Mix and serve as garnish or as a salad dressing. Just before serving, add the set-aside zest.

Black Olive/Tomato Relish

1 cup black Kalamata olives

1 clove garlic

1 medium tomato quartered

¼ olive oil

Place olives, garlic, and tomatoes in food processor and puree. With the motor running, drizzle in the olive oil in a constant stream. Remove and serve as needed. Can be refrigerated in covered container for a week.

Non-dairy Pesto

1 cup fresh basil leaves

½ cup pine nuts

2 cloves garlic

¼ cup olive oil

Combine basil, pine nuts, and garlic in food processor and puree.
With the motor running, add olive oil in a steady stream until thickened.

Lemon Mayonnaise

1 whole egg

2 T fresh lemon juice

Pinch of salt

½ tsp dry mustard

½ cup olive oil

Lemon zest for garnish

Combine egg, lemon juice, mustard, and salt in food processor fitted with blade. Puree until ingredients are incorporated. Stop. Whirl and, with the motor running, slowly add the oil in a drizzle. Your mayonnaise will be thinner than the commercial brand but lighter tasting and so much better for you.

Aioli

1 whole egg

3 cloves fresh garlic

Pinch of salt

1 T fresh lemon juice

½ cup olive oil

Combine egg, salt, garlic, and lemon juice in food processor and puree. Stop. Begin again and, while the motor is running slowly drizzle the olive oil into egg mixture until you have a lighter-than-mayonnaise consistency.

▶ To make basil aioli, add a handful of fresh basil leaves before adding oil.

▶ To make cilantro aioli, add a handful of cilantro before adding oil.

Canned Goods

Nutrient-dense legumes

Black beans

Cannellini beans (white kidney beans)

Kidney beans

Baby lima beans

Garbanzo beans (chickpeas)

Oils and Vinegars

Extra-virgin olive oil

Sesame oil

Rice wine vinegar

Balsamic vinegar

Red wine vinegar

Canola oil

Freezer Supplies

Blueberries, raspberries, blackberries

Fava beans

Edamame

Easy Tomato Sauce

3 medium whole tomatoes
1 clove garlic
5 large leaves of fresh basil (or 2 tsp dried basil)
¼ cup olive oil
1 tsp lemon juice
Pinch of salt and cracked pepper to taste

Place whole unpeeled tomatoes in food processor with garlic and lemon juice. Puree until tomatoes are well blended. With the motor running, slowly add the olive oil. Taste and add pinch of salt and cracked pepper if desired.

This quick little all-purpose garnish stores well in a lidded jar in the refrigerator for three days. Use it to top or garnish pastas, soups, vegetables, pizzas, fish, or vegetables. Makes 1 cup.

Getting Started

*Brain-healthy food options can inspire culinary creativity.
The deeper, the richer, the more colorful the fruits and
vegetables, the more likely they are to be what your
brain needs.*

Although the cuisine we've been describing is obviously attractive to people with neurodegenerative diseases, it is also a healthy alternative for anyone who is interested in preventive health care.

When we understand the benefits of changing our shopping lists from processed foods and bad fats to the fresh and colorful options that are actually good for us and our children, we are ready to positively influence a whole generation of diners—one family at a time.

That change might require a shift in lifestyle. Begin gradually by thinking about what you purchase, how you prepare ingredients, and how you eat your food. Once you begin that process, you're on the road to mindful eating.

We do not suggest that you be a slave to perfection. Just get started by cooking with flavorful seeds and beans, whole grains and nuts, and an extensive array of antioxidant fruits and vegetables. Add occasional fish and pasta to your repertoire—using sauces made with garlic and olive oil—and more deeply colored vegetables. Eventually, you might just discover your body craves an afternoon snack of something as simple and nutritious as richly flavored toasted walnuts or pecans accompanied by a dark purple plum.

Start thinking like a neuroprotective detective. The deeper, the richer, the more colorful the fruits and vegetables, the more likely they are to be what your brain needs. A good example is the deep red color and rich sweet taste of the blood orange!

We have limited the number of dessert recipes because we almost always finish our meals with a salad! We have also discovered that fresh fruit is an entirely satisfying dessert. We got hooked on the fruit habit in Mexico, where we could pick grapefruit and oranges from the trees every day during the winter. But even at home, we can find good fresh fruit all year long.

Summer fruits grown locally are abundant in the Northwest. In July, we eat Rainier and red cherries and strawberries. August is for plums, raspberries, and black berries. September brings pears, blueberries, Asian pears, apples, and figs.

Why Salmon?

Why *wild* salmon? Why not the cheaper farmed salmon? There are important differences between the two. First of all, we do not recommend daily consumption of fish, but when you do, try to eat fish that is known to provide the proper nutrients.

The body cannot manufacture essential omega-3 oils. They must be obtained from food sources, such as canola oil, flaxseed oil, some legumes (beans and peas that grow inside pods), and wild ocean salmon.

Fish has often been classified as "brain food," and with good reason. The brain contains more than 60 percent fat. The fatty acids found in fish, such as salmon, are essential to optimal functioning our brain cells.

Wild salmon is the best choice, primarily because their ocean diet consists of a variety of aquatic organisms. Wild salmon contain high levels of essential omega-3 oils. Most farm-raised salmon are fed an unnatural diet of high-fat feed primarily made of soybean/wheat meal combined with ground-up fish parts, plus antibiotics. Most farmed fish retain the man-made chemical contaminants of their feed in their fatty tissues, and they have tiny amounts of omega-3 oils to offer. In addition, farm-raised salmon contain much higher levels of pro-inflammatory omega-6 oils.

Wild Pacific king salmon, Coho, sockeye, or Copper River are the most beneficial choices.

Other safe and sustainable fish include: U.S. farmed tilapia, flounder, sable fish, black cod, Dungeness crab, stone crab, Pacific halibut, farmed bay scallops, Oregon pink shrimp, haddock, and farm-raised trout. Most canned salmon is wild; check the label to be sure.

SALMON RECIPES

On days when Mike comes into the kitchen with a new basket of freshly chopped fruitwood chips, I get the message. It's time to purchase a grand filet of fresh wild king salmon, which are readily available year-round in our area. We are also fortunate to have old apple, wild plum, and pear trees on our property, and luckily these trees require yearly pruning. One small 3-inch chunk of fruit wood will adequately flavor a 3-pound salmon filet.

Smoke-Cooked Wild King Salmon with Mango Salsa

This recipe is designed with elegant leftovers in mind; it can be used the day of grilling, or with leftovers that have been carefully covered and refrigerated the previous day.

Salmon grilled beside coals with smoking wood chips will give you the most delicate and fulfilling taste sensation; it's an effort you'll not regret. This method of cooking salmon always triggers Mike's taste buds well before he sits down to eat.

To Grill

Use a chimney to start charcoal—no starter fluid!!!

½ cup, or one 3-inch chunk of light fruit wood—pear, plum, or apple
Soak wood in water to cover while you dress the salmon, for about ½ hour.
1–3 pound filet of wild salmon

Dressing

2 T olive oil	Freshly cracked pepper
2 cloves garlic, finely chopped	Zest of whole lemon
2 tsp sea salt	Juice of half lemon, about 1 T

Top the flesh of the salmon filet with ingredients above and let rest until coals are ready. When all coals are burning, pour them into one end of fire pit or grill and place soaked wood chips on top of fire. Place a heavy griddle or cookie sheet on top of the grill, directly over the flames. Brush canola oil lightly over the grill. Then place the salmon skin side down on the grill next to the cookie sheet (but not directly over the coals), the fish will cook from the smoke and indirect heat. Close the lid, so that the fruit wood smoke can work its magic.

Cook salmon 10 minutes per pound. Do not turn. Remove salmon from grill. Remember that the fish will continue to cook after removing it from the heat, so gauge your preferred doneness, tenderness, and succulence accordingly. If you do not have access to a grill, you can steam, poach, or bake your salmon in the oven.

Mango Salsa
Ripe mango (or three fresh peaches), peeled and chopped
2 tsp ginger root, chopped
1 clove garlic, chopped
2 T red onion, minced
2 T Jalapeno pepper, chopped
2 T cilantro, chopped
Pinch of cinnamon

Combine above ingredients then add dressing.

Dressing
2 T olive oil   2 tsp fresh lime juice
1 T red wine vinegar

Combine all ingredients and mix.

Vegetable Lasagna with Salmon
Not everybody has the desire or the time to make their own pasta, but once you've tried it, you might think twice about going to the store to buy spaghetti, fettuccini, or lasagna noodles. Homemade noodles are fresh, silken, fast, economical, fun to make, and always a hit! But either fresh-prepared from the store or dried pasta will make a good substitute.

Bechamel Sauce (White Sauce)
3 T butter substitute (such as Smart Balance or Earth Balance; Earth Balance is completely non-dairy)
3 T flour
2 cups unflavored soy or almond milk
1 scraping of fresh nutmeg or a pinch of dried
Salt to taste

Melt the butter in a heavy-bottomed saucepan. Add the flour and whisk quickly to blend butter and flour. Add soy (or almond) milk and continue whisking over medium heat until sauce has thickened. Taste and add salt and nutmeg. Taste again and let rest while you prepare the lasagna layers. Makes 2 cups.

Lasagna Noodles
If you use pre-made pasta, try to use noodles prepared from whole wheat (preferably durum wheat) and cook according to directions. This recipe makes 20 lasagna noodles.

3 cups of flour
4 eggs
1 T canola oil

Pour flour onto countertop, or into a wide bowl and make a well in the center of the flour. Crack eggs into the well. Using your fingers, begin gathering bits of the flour into the center of the well, blending egg with flour a little bit at a time until flour and eggs are completely incorporated. Then knead the dough just lightly until you have a well-formed ball.

Set up your noodle maker, following directions for lasagna noodles, and cutting them as directed.

In a 3-quart pot boil water with 1 T of canola oil and add noodles (either homemade or store-bought). Boil for 5 minutes; drain water off and refill pot with warm water to cover noodles until you're ready for assembly of lasagna.

Layers

Salmon with Roasted Red Pepper Layer

Flake 2 cups precooked salmon and toss with strips of 1 whole Roasted Red
  Pepper (Pantry, page 94).

Mushroom Layer

2 cups mushrooms of any combination—shitake, oyster, morels, or white button; wash mushrooms and cut oyster mushrooms loose from the base.

½ cup chicken or mushroom bouillon. (I use McCormick chicken bouillon
  cubes, or organic Better Than Bouillon mushroom base [1 tsp to 8 ounces
  of water]).

3 T sweet onion, minced

2 scrapings of fresh nutmeg or ½ tsp dry

½ tsp dried tarragon or a 1 T of fresh tarragon

¼ cup dry white wine

Sprinkling of salt

2 grinds of freshly cracked pepper

Slice morel, shitake, and button mushrooms. In a heavy skillet, bring
bouillon to a boil, then add onions and mushrooms. Simmer until mushrooms
are slightly tender. Add wine and tarragon, and simmer another 5 minutes.
Add salt, pepper, and nutmeg. Stir and remove from heat. Let rest until ready
to assemble lasagna.

Spinach/Leek Layer

1 whole leek, cut down the center and thoroughly washed then chopped in half
  inch slices

11 ounces fresh spinach leaves washed, stems removed, and chopped

2 T canola oil

2 cloves garlic, chopped

¼ cup fresh parsley, chopped

Fresh lemon juice

Grating of nutmeg, salt, and cracked pepper

Heat 2 T canola oil in heavy skillet and sauté leeks with 2 cloves of chopped garlic until leeks are wilted. Squeeze fresh lemon juice over leeks. Remove leeks from pan and set aside. To the same pan, add spinach and cook down to about 1 cup. Mix leeks, spinach, and chopped parsley together, season with nutmeg, lemon juice, and a little salt and pepper to taste.

Lasagna Assembly

Preheat oven to 350 degrees. Taste each combination and add salt and pepper to taste before assembly. Remove enough noodles from water to make bottom layer in a 9 × 13 lasagna pan. One suggested order: noodles, spinach/leek, white sauce, another layer of noodles, mushrooms, white sauce, noodles, flaked salmon with sliced roasted red pepper, a final layer of noodles, topped with remainder of white sauce.

Cover lasagna with waxed paper then foil and bake at 350 degrees for 35 minutes.

To serve: Top each serving of lasagna with 1 T of Black Olive/Tomato Relish (Pantry, page 98). Garnish with a good grating of lemon zest!

Salmon/Tilapia Chowder with Aioli

1 pound fresh salmon, cut into 1-inch chunks (if you don't have salmon, substitute flounder)

¼ pound fresh tilapia, cut to bite size

2 cups Tomato Base (Pantry, page 96)

2 T olive oil

1 15-ounce can cannellini beans, drained and rinsed

1 T lovage, or 4 stalks celery with leaves, chopped

1 cup dry white wine

2 tsp turmeric

1 T fresh thyme or 1 tsp dried

3 medium potatoes, peeled and chopped into ½-inch cubes (I like Yukon Gold or other yellow potatoes but you can use any good potato)

1 cup sweet potato, peeled and cut into ½-inch cubes

1 cup carrots, sliced
1 cube chicken bouillon
1 dozen black Kalamata olives
2 cups water
Freshly cracked pepper

For the Garnish
1 recipe Aioli (Pantry, page 99)
2 T capers
1 roasted red pepper, cut in thin strips (instructions Pantry, page 94)
Lemon juice

In a large soup kettle, add 2 T olive oil and sauté potatoes, with the sweet potatoes, stirring until coated. Add Tomato Base, turmeric, thyme, beans, white wine, chicken bouillon, and water. Reduce to moderate heat for 25 minutes or until potatoes are tender. Add salmon (or substitute), tilapia, and olives. Stir and let simmer for another 3–5 minutes, until fish is flaky. Salt and pepper to taste. Adjust seasoning. Serves four.

Garnishes to Serve with Salmon

Roast a red pepper and cut into long strips. Serve chowder with a healthy dollop of aioli sauce and garnish with a few strings of roasted red pepper, capers, and a squeeze of fresh lemon.

Here are some ideas for salmon-compatible ingredients to roll inside rice paper wrappers (or tapioca flour wrappers). Experiment to discover what other antioxidant ingredients might be successful collaborators.

Fresh Veggie/Salmon Spring Rolls

8-inch rice flour wrappers (3 rolls per person; I use tapioca flour wrappers. They are less frustrating to roll and they stick together better than rice wrappers.)

6 leaves dark Bibb lettuce, one per roll. (Bibb leaves are supple and easy to wrap.)

1 cup grilled or otherwise precooked fresh salmon

Mangos, peaches, or pears, peeled and cut into thin slices

Half an English cucumber, thinly sliced

Clover sprouts or other fresh sprouts

1 T lime peel, cut into tiny strips—you must try this!

1 T ginger root, peeled and finely chopped

1 avocado, thinly sliced

1 cup carrots, grated

Arrange all ingredients (except wrappers) on a large platter in separate mounds. Bring water to a boil, for softening the wrappers. In a deep, heat-resistant plate or bowl, pour 1 inch of boiling water. Place one wrapper at a time into the hot water and swirl around until soft—about 10 seconds. (You may need to reheat water occasionally to keep it hot enough to soften all the wrappers.)

Place softened wrapper on a plate and arrange contents, first placing lettuce leaf on top of wrapper, then adding salmon and vegetables in the center of the lettuce. Fold one side of the wrapper over the filling and tuck in the ends as you roll, forming a tight package. It gets easier and tidier, the more you roll. Serves two.

Dipping Sauce

1 T fresh lime juice

1 T rice wine vinegar

2 T fish sauce (I use Tiparos, but you can find different brands of fish sauce in some groceries and most Asian markets)

1 T sugar

3 T water

½ tsp red chili pepper; if fresh, chop it, if dried, crush it

½ cup shredded carrots

Combine sugar, water, lime, and vinegar. Whisk until sugar is dissolved. Add fish sauce and chopped or crushed peppers. Add carrots. This sauce can also be used as a marinade for shrimp. Serve sauce in individual bowls at the table, with watermelon or other seasonal fruit for dessert. Serves two.

Salmon Cakes

No salmon? Substitute flounder, Oregon pink shrimp or Dungeness crab. These little gems are easy to prepare, forgiving, and versatile. They can be formed into patties, covered, and refrigerated, even overnight. They will cooperate if company is late and you have to re-heat them. Makes four 3-inch patties.

2 cups cooked and flaked salmon or substitute

½ cup home made mayonnaise (page 98)

1 cup ground white bread crumbs

Juice of half a lemon

1 T shredded onion

1 egg

1 tsp sesame oil

A pinch of salt

2 cracks of ground pepper

2 T canola oil

1 T fresh dill or fennel leaves

For Garnish

½ avocado   Lemon zest

1 dozen blueberries   Dill or fennel

In a medium-sized mixing bowl, combine half the bread crumbs (reserve other half for coating) and remainder of ingredients except canola oil and fresh dill or fennel. Mix together and shape into patties. Dredge patties through remaining bread crumbs to coat. At this stage, you can cover and refrigerate patties up to over-night, until you're ready to cook them.

To cook salmon cakes: Heat 2 T canola oil in a heavy frying pan. Over medium heat, fry salmon patties about 7 minutes on each side. These patties will keep again for an hour or so (if necessary), and can be reheated in a 350-degree oven until warm throughout—about 12 minutes.

Serve each patty on a single leaf of dark lettuce and dress with red sauce.

Red Dressing
¼ cup chili sauce
¼ cup lemon/ mayonnaise (recipe page 98)
1 fresh tomato, finely chopped
1 T capers
1 T sweet onion, shredded
Juice of half a lemon

Mix all ingredients. Spoon sauce over one half the salmon patty, top with lemon zest. Garnish by arranging three to five slices of avocado along the sauced edge of the lettuce and drop blueberries inside the lettuce leaf. Sprinkle dill or fennel over all and add a zest of lemon. The surprise entrance of blue-berries will charm and delight you!

Winter Nights: Soups and More

THE ORIGIN OF SOUP

The tradition of combining varied and nutritious, easily digested, soothing ingredients into a great big cooking pot and calling the outcome *soup*, *chowder*, *stew*, or *potage* is as old as the history of cooking. Soups evolved differently according to each culture and have been prescribed for invalids since ancient times. *Restoratifs* (bouillons and consommés), believed to restore the body and the soul, were the first items served in French restaurants in 18th-century Paris.

A WORD ABOUT DRIED BEANS

It's worth the time and effort to learn the correct cooking procedure for dried beans. They are economical and packed with nutrients, and we need them to be at their best.

The black bean is smaller than other beans, and the hole in its bottom is so small that it takes longer for moisture to enter the bean. The older the bean, the longer the cooking time. Older black beans can take as long as 2 hours to cook. So, your cooking technique must be adjusted accordingly.

Marjoram

First, a word about an extraordinarily aromatic but often neglected herb that can be successfully used in many hearty soup recipes.

With a delicate floral aroma and layers of complexity including a hint of balsam, sweet knotted marjoram is an unheralded, but nevertheless magnificent "player," worthy of space in this cookbook. The ancient Romans believed that marjoram represented happiness, and Hippocrates included it in many of his medical treatises.

Contributing its own antioxidant properties, marjoram is compelling and the most interesting when its flowers and leaves are used while the herb is still supple and fresh. It is often referred to as "oregano," but marjoram is actually a member of the mint family. The difference between oregano and marjoram is obvious to the eye, the nose, the palate, and—most of all—to the spirit. The sweet piney taste of the buds just before they pop open is exhilarating. If you don't have access to fresh marjoram, the dried herb "holds its own" more successfully than other dried herbs, and it gets along well with other food flavors when combined in dishes.

The first step in cooking dried beans is to pick through the beans and discard any little stones or twigs. Then, for best results, pre-soak the beans overnight; this is especially important for black beans.

To pre-soak beans overnight, cover them with 2 inches of water and allow plenty of room for expansion. The next day, drain off the water and cover the beans with fresh water before cooking.

Next—and this applies to cooking all dried beans—do not add salt or acidic ingredients such as lemon, vinegar, wine, or tomatoes until the beans are finished cooking or nearly done, otherwise they can toughen.

Finally, if your diners are concerned with flatulence, add summer savory to the recipe. Now I think we're ready for a bean recipe!

Three-Bean Chili

½ cup dried black beans or 1 15-ounce can

½ cup dried cannellini beans or 1 15-ounce can

½ cup dried pinto beans or 1 15-ounce can

If using dried beans: Soak beans overnight, using a separate pot for the black beans. Drain water off, cover with fresh water, and cook until the beans are tender, about 40 minutes.

3 T olive oil

1 cup sweet onion, chopped

½ cup celery, chopped, or 1 T fresh lovage, chopped, if available (lovage is a large perennial herb in the carrot family that tastes like intense celery with hints of allspice)

½ cup carrots, chopped

2 tsp turmeric

1 tsp cumin seed

2 tsp ground coriander seeds (smash seeds with the back of a big spoon or grind in coffee grinder)

4 cloves garlic, chopped

2 14-ounce cans seasoned tomatoes

1 T oregano

2 T rosemary

1 T thyme

1 T chili powder

1 T summer savory

½ tsp cinnamon

1 T dark cocoa powder (optional, but contains antioxidants and great flavor)

3 cups organic mushroom or vegetable broth

½ cup hearty red wine

Salt and cracked pepper

Garnish

Chunky salsa (page 161) and lime wedges

Using a large heavy-bottomed soup kettle, heat 2 T olive oil and add the chopped onions. Sauté the onions, stirring until soft, but not toasted or over-cooked. Add chopped garlic, herbs, and spices. Stir to mix. Add carrots, celery (or lovage), and stir until coated. Add bouillon, wine, water, cooked or canned beans, and tomatoes. Simmer over medium-low heat for 1 hour *or* transfer to a slow cooker and cook on low for 3 hours. Salt and pepper to taste. Adjust seasonings.

To serve: Top each serving with chunky salsa and a wedge of lime. Pass bowls of chopped cilantro and more salsa. Makes 8 cups.

Butternut Squash Soup

What a beautiful vegetable! Squash is commonly considered a vegetable in cooking, but actually squash is a fruit, botanically speaking, because the squash is the receptacle for the seeds of the plant. You'd never know it by its outward appearance, but inside you will discover the most alluring, luscious hues of orange—squash is also loaded with beta-carotene.

1 whole 2–3-pound butternut squash
3 cups water with one chicken bouillon cube or equal amount of prepared
    stock
1 thin slice of ginger root
½ tsp cinnamon
1 tsp turmeric

Garnish

4 T plain fat-free yogurt with lime

Lime zest

Saffron threads (Optional; don't fret about saffron, it's very expensive, but if someone gives it to you for a gift, this would be a beautiful way to use it.)

Cut top and bottom off the squash, then cut in half lengthwise and remove seeds. Using a vegetable peeler, peel the squash, making two passes to get to the rich orange color. Cut into 1-inch chunks. In a stock pot, bring the chicken stock to a boil and add squash. Simmer on medium-high heat 20 minutes or until squash is tender.

Using a slotted spoon, transfer squash to a food processor or blender. Add ginger root, cinnamon, and turmeric. Puree until very smooth. Transfer squash back to stock pot. Stir over medium heat to warm.

Garnish each serving of soup with 1 T of lime-flavored yogurt (recipe below) topped with a few threads of saffron. Serves six.

Lime-flavored Yogurt
3 ounces of plain fat-free yogurt   Zest of one lime
1 tsp lime juice

Mix ingredients together.

Other Garnish Options
Drizzle pureed Roasted Red Pepper (Pantry, page 94) over the soup. Or, try adding peeled and chopped fresh pear bits with toasted hazelnuts to the finished soup.

Quick and Beautiful: Potage for Two
4 medium potatoes, peeled and quartered
2 cups chicken bouillon
1 roasted red pepper, seeded and cut in half (instructions for roasting, Pantry, page 94)
1 T onion, chopped
1 clove garlic, minced
½ tsp turmeric
1 T fresh tarragon or ½ tsp dried
Optional: Garnish of 2 T Olive Tower (Pantry, pages 96–97)

Bring chicken stock to boil; add potatoes, onion, and garlic. Cook over medium heat until potatoes are tender. Using a slotted spoon, transfer potatoes, onions, and garlic with some bouillon to food processor. Add roasted red pepper, tarragon, and turmeric. Blend until very smooth but not sticky, adding more chicken stock if necessary. Transfer back to cooking pot and reheat with any remaining chicken stock. This soup should be thick but not as thick as mashed potatoes. If soup needs thinning, add more bouillon to your desired consistency. Add salt and freshly cracked pepper to taste. Serve with 1 T Black Olive Tower (Pantry, pages 96–97) in the center and a squeeze of lemon juice.

Spinach Soup

Mike made this recipe for lunch one day when I was sick. It's amazingly simple and very good!

1 pound fresh spinach washed and dried
2 cups chicken bouillon (2 cups water plus 1 bouillon cube)
2 gratings of fresh nutmeg
Lemon zest

Set up food processor with pureeing blade. In a large skillet, combine spinach with 1 cup of bouillon. Cook down until spinach is wilted, then transfer to food processor. Puree the spinach until very smooth. Transfer to a medium soup pot and add remaining bouillon and nutmeg. Heat. Garnish with lemon zest. Serves 2.

Mushroom Soup

2 T butter substitute (Earth Balance or Smart Balance)
2 T flour
½ pound white button mushrooms, finely chopped
2 cups water
2 tsp mushroom or vegetable bouillon
1 T fresh tarragon leaves or 1 tsp dried

2 gratings fresh nutmeg
4 T toasted sliced almonds
Salt and cracked pepper to taste

Melt butter substitute in medium-sized saucepan. Whisk in flour and mix over heat. Add water with bouillon and whisk until smooth and thick. Add mushrooms, tarragon, and nutmeg. Reduce heat to simmer until completely heated about 10 minutes. Serve soup topped with toasted almonds. Serves two.

Brainy Minestrone Soup

In Italy, the test of successful minestrone (aside from the taste) is whether your spoon can stand on its own in the bowl!

This is a great recipe to make in a slow cooker.

½ cup dried pinto beans, or one 15-ounce can, rinsed and drained
½ cup dried cannellini beans or one 15-ounce can, drained
½ cup dried or frozen fava beans

If using dried beans, soak overnight. Rinse beans and add fresh water to cover. Cook 40 minutes or until tender. Drain.

4 cloves garlic, chopped
½ cup onion, chopped
2 T olive oil
1 cup celery, chopped
2 tsp turmeric
1 T fresh rosemary
2 tsp fresh marjoram or ½ tsp dried marjoram
½ cup parsley, chopped
2 tsp dried basil
4 cups Tomato Base (Pantry, page 96)
3 cups mushroom or vegetable stock
2 carrots, chopped
2 medium zucchini, sliced

1 cup hearty red wine Burgundy or Beaujolais
2 cups cooked penne pasta, or other pasta of your choice
Garnish with ½ cup Pesto (Pantry, page 98)

In a slow cooker, combine stock, cooked or canned beans, carrots, Tomato Base, celery, garlic, marjoram, turmeric, rosemary, parsley, basil, and wine. Slow cook 4 hours on low heat.

Thirty minutes before serving, sauté zucchini in olive oil until just tender. Add zucchini and pasta to the pot. Adjust salt and freshly cracked pepper to taste.

Top each serving with a dollop of pesto. Pass extra pesto at the table. Serves six.

Asparagus Soup

½ pound fresh asparagus
2 T sweet onion, minced
3 T butter substitute (Earth Balance or Smart Balance)
3 T flour
2 cups chicken or vegetable bouillon
½ tsp nutmeg, freshly grated
Salt and cracked pepper to taste

Wash and trim fresh asparagus. Bring bouillon to a boil with onion. Add asparagus and cook until just tender. Transfer to food processor and puree until smooth.

Make a roux by melting butter substitute in a saucepan over medium heat. Add flour to butter while whisking to incorporate. Add bouillon and pureed asparagus and whisk to blend. Add nutmeg and heat. Garnish with a grating of lemon zest.

Tomato or broccoli soup

Substitute cooked and pureed broccoli or 1 cup of pureed Tomato Base (Pantry, page 96). Serves two.

Lemon-Lentil Soup

1 cup lentils

6 cups water

1 medium sweet onion, peeled and quartered

3 large cloves garlic, halved

1 medium potato, peeled and quartered

2 tsp ground flax seeds

2 carrots or ½ cup, peeled and sliced

1 tsp turmeric

1 tsp fresh marjoram or a pinch of dried

¼ cup parsley, chopped

Juice of whole lemon

Salt and cracked pepper to taste

Garnish

Lemon zest

1 T capers

In a large cooking pot, combine lentils, water, onion, garlic, potato, carrots, turmeric, flax seeds, marjoram, and parsley. Simmer for 1 hour. Transfer beans and vegetables to food processor and puree until smooth, adding additional stock as needed. Transfer puree back to cooking pot. Stir soup while heating. Add lemon juice. Add salt and cracked pepper to taste.

Garnish with lemon zest and capers, or try nasturtium flowers and buds. These zesty little characters look like a party and taste like capers, but without the brine. Serves four.

Gaspacho—Chilled Soup

Here's one for summertime!

Gaspacho is simply good, refreshing, and energizing. There's no mystery with this one. Gaspacho looks you straight in the eye and let's you know where it stands, and what it has to offer.

2 small cucumbers, peeled, seeded, and chopped, or one entire English cucumber, chopped

3 tomatoes, peeled (instructions Pantry, pages 93–94) and chopped

1 green pepper, seeded and chopped

1 small sweet onion, minced

3 cloves garlic, chopped

¼ cup fresh basil, chopped

1 T parsley, chopped

1 16-ounce can V-8 juice

3 T olive oil

1 T red wine vinegar

Salt and cracked pepper to taste

Extra fresh basil for garnish

Combine chopped vegetables with garlic, basil, olive oil, and vinegar in a large bowl. Pour in V-8 juice. Stir and taste. Add freshly cracked pepper and chill. If soup becomes too thick, stir in more V-8 juice just before serving.

Garnish with lemon zest and more chopped fresh basil. Serves four.

Eggplant with Turmeric Yogurt

Eggplant is a nutritional powerhouse: it's high in dietary fiber, folate, potassium, manganese, vitamins C, K, and B_6, thiamin, niacin, pantothenic acid, magnesium, phosphorus, and copper. The skin contains *nasunin*, a powerful antioxidant. Eggplant is also low is saturated fat, sodium, and cholesterol, and high in antioxidants.

This is a wonderful-tasting entrée with perfect cooking juices for sopping with fresh warm bread.

1 medium eggplant, unpeeled and sliced into ½-inch rounds (about 12 slices)
4 T salt
½ cup olive oil
1 medium sweet onion, sliced into ¼-inch rounds
4 medium tomatoes
1½ cups plain fat-free yogurt
2 tsp turmeric

Place eggplant slices in a large bowl. Sprinkle salt over all slices of eggplant and let stand for 1 hour to extract moisture. Rinse salt from eggplant and wipe dry with paper towel.

In a medium bowl, mix yogurt and turmeric together to make a pale yellow blend.

In a large, heavy skillet, heat 4 T olive oil. When oil is hot, begin sautéing eggplant slices, adding olive oil as needed, until all eggplant slices are golden. You probably will use the entire ½ cup of olive oil.

Arrange layers in ovenproof 4–5-inch deep casserole. Begin with a layer of eggplant, then a layer of tomato slices, then half the yogurt, then a layer of onions. Begin again with eggplant, continuing on until final layer of yogurt.

Cover and bake in 350 oven 45 minutes.

Serve with warm pita bread and a small bowl of olive/tomato relish (recipe on page 98). Generously serves two.

Pita Bread with Macha Green Tea for Sopping and Mopping

These individual servings of lovely fresh bread will provide hours of happy "sopping." Pita bread is just what you'll need to capture every drop of juice and olive oil in the bottom of your bowl. Pita bread is readily available in many stores, but you may want to try making your own using this recipe.

1 cup lukewarm water

2 tsp active dry yeast

2½ cups all-purpose flour (optional: mix in 1 tsp powdered Macha green tea for more antioxidants)

Additional flour for baking pan

½ tsp salt

2½ T olive oil

In a small bowl, combine water and 2 T oil with yeast and let stand for 5 minutes. In a large bread bowl, combine 2 cups flour, tea, and salt. Make a well in the center of the flour and stir in the yeast. Mix together until it becomes a compact dough.

Place dough on a floured surface and knead in remaining ½ cup flour for 10 minutes, until dough is smooth, elastic, and not sticky. Shape into a ball and place in a bowl that has been rubbed with olive oil. Cover with a clean towel and let rise for 1–2 hours until doubled. Punch the dough down and let rest for 10 minutes.

Preheat oven to 450 degrees and place a baking sheet or heavy griddle on the middle shelf of the oven to heat up.

Cut dough into ten pieces and shape each piece into a small ball.

This next step creates the puff in the center of your pita, if you want to use the bread for sandwiches. If you prefer flat bread, leave out this step: Flatten each piece with your fingers making a 3–4-inch round.

Fold dough, taking the left side to the center, then the right side, then the bottom half to the center, then the top half. Press into the center and turn piece over with seam side down on counter. Repeat for all eight pieces. Continue recipe as for flat breads.

Let pieces rest for 10 minutes. Using a rolling pin, roll each piece flat to about 5 inches in diameter. Sprinkle a little flour on the baking sheet in the oven and begin transferring the dough rounds onto the hot baking sheet. Bake for 8–10 minutes or until bread is either puffed in the center or toasted on the bottom or both.

These breads will stay warm if they are gently wrapped in a clean towel. Best to serve them warm. If you have to reheat the pitas, do so for 3–4 minutes in a preheated oven or 15 seconds in a microwave. They will cooperate beautifully. Makes about ten 4-inch pitas.

Make ahead of time: You can prepare the pita dough through the first 1–2-hour rising, punch it down, and store it in the refrigerator for up to 24 hours in a zipper-close plastic bag until you are ready to continue preparation.

Another option: Substitute all-purpose flour with a mixture of 1 cup of whole wheat flour to 1½ cups all-purpose flour.

Classic Ratatouille

1 medium eggplant, peeled and cut into ½-inch slices
1 medium tender zucchini, unpeeled and cut into cubes
4 medium tomatoes, peeled (see Pantry, pages 93–94)
½ cup onion, chopped
1 whole green bell pepper, cut into ½-inch pieces
4 cloves garlic, minced
¼ cup fresh basil, scissor-cut in strips
½ tsp turmeric
½ cup olive oil
Salt and pepper to taste
1 T per serving of pine nuts
1 recipe Aioli (Pantry, page 99)
1 recipe Pesto (Pantry, page 98)

Preheat oven to 350 degrees. Place sliced eggplant on paper towel and salt each piece. Let stand for 30 minutes. Pat dry and set aside.

In a large, heavy-bottomed skillet, heat 2 T olive oil. Add chopped eggplant and stir with a wooden spoon until tender, adding more oil if needed. Remove eggplant to a 2-quart oven-proof casserole. Add more olive oil to skillet and sauté zucchini until almost tender. Add zucchini to eggplant and continue sautéing onions and green pepper. Mix all ingredients in casserole and add chopped garlic, turmeric, and half the chopped basil.

Cover casserole with lid or foil and bake for 40 minutes. Just before serving, stir in remaining basil; salt and pepper to taste. Sprinkle ratatouille with pine nuts and serve with little bowls of pesto and aioli. Makes two to four servings.

Quick Version "Ratatouille," The Movie Star

My interpretation of this faster-cooking version of the classic recipe is similar to the one presented in the popular movie, "Ratatouille."

The trick with this adaptation is to use thinly sliced vegetables for swift baking. You will need an 8-inch round pizza pan (or other round baking pan with edges), a round of freezer or parchment paper cut to the shape of the pan, and a lid or plate that fits tightly over the pan.

½ recipe Pesto (Pantry, page 98)
1 recipe Aioli (Pantry, page 99)
1½ cup Tomato Base (Pantry, page 96)
1 medium zucchini, very thinly sliced
1 medium Japanese eggplant with skin on, thinly sliced. Use the smaller, longer
    Japanese eggplant to match the size of zucchini.
1 small Walla Walla (or other sweet onion), thinly sliced
1 green pepper, thinly sliced into rings
2 T olive oil

Arrange vegetables in an overlapping pattern around the edge of the baking pan, alternating one slice of eggplant, then one slice zucchini, green pepper slice, onion slice, until all the vegetables are arranged. Drizzle the vegetables with 2 T of olive oil. Sprinkle with salt and grind fresh pepper over all vegetables. Cover vegetables with circle of freezer paper and cover with a plate to compress the vegetables while they bake. Bake at 350 degrees for 25 minutes.

Puree the Tomato Base in the food processor until smooth. Heat the sauce.

To serve: Pour a pool of hot tomato sauce onto the center of a plate. Transfer half the vegetables onto the red sauce, creating a kind of leaning tower. Drizzle with Aioli and decorate with pesto. Serves two.

A Word About Turmeric

Many of the recipes in this chapter incorporate the powerful ingredient turmeric, an antioxidant spice "star." It shines. It glows without overwhelming other ingredients. Rather turmeric enhances ingredients by deepening individual strengths and flavors. The taste of turmeric by itself is a subtle and delicate orange rind and ginger.

Curcumin is the active ingredient in turmeric. The medicinal properties of this Indian spice have been the focus of study for centuries.

Primarily known to be an anti-inflammatory, turmeric is proving to be beneficial in the treatment of other health conditions, from cancer to Alzheimer's disease. It may aid in fat metabolism and help in weight management, and it's inexpensive!

There are numerous reasons to add turmeric to your diet. With so many opportunities to enhance other ingredients, you'll wonder why you waited so long to get to know turmeric.

Simple Green Salad

Many people enjoy a simple, fresh salad dressing recipe, rather than using processed bottled dressings.

1 head red or green leaf, Bibb, mixed baby salad greens, or romaine lettuce, washed and dried

1 clove fresh garlic, chopped
1 T fresh tarragon
1 T balsamic vinegar
2 T olive oil
Pinch of salt
Zest of half a lemon

Fruit Options

½ Honeycrisp or other firm apple, peeled and thinly sliced; fresh ripe pear, seeded, unpeeled, and thinly sliced; or, try a scant handful of reconstituted dried sour cherries or fresh in-season cherries. To reconstitute dried cherries, pour boiling water over dried cherries; wait 5 minutes, drain and squeeze the liquid from the fruit, then add to the salad.

Nut Options

¼ cup toasted walnuts, pecans, or hazelnuts—or a combination of all of these, slightly crushed. Or, use pumpkin or sunflower seeds.

Combine vinegar and oil in a large salad bowl. Sprinkle salt over the oil, and then add chopped garlic, sliced apples, and cherries. (If you're using pears, wait until the last minute to add them or they may get mushy)

Add washed and dried lettuce, nuts, and fresh tarragon to the bowl. Do not toss salad until you're ready to serve. Of course, you can serve salad whenever you wish. Usually, when it's "just us," we have salad for dessert.

Just before tossing the salad, add the toasted, slightly crushed nuts and the pear slices. Top with lemon zest. The dressing is just waiting at the bottom of the bowl, flavoring the apples slices but not wilting the lettuce. Just before serving, toss the salad gently with two big spoons. Serves two.

Slaws

The word "slaw" comes from the Dutch, meaning salad. Ingredients for exciting slaws are versatile and available year-round. You can create a slaw from a variety of cabbages and root plants, and flavor your salad with herbs, nuts, seeds, and oils to suit your taste.

Beets are loaded with nutrients, including folate, manganese, and potassium. Cooking beets releases a rich, earthy flavor. Beets come in various colors: common red beets, golden beets, and pink and white striated Chioggia beets. My favorite use for beets is in salads, but we have some other fun options to offer.

Beet Slaw with Mint and Red Onion

1 medium fresh beet
Bermuda onion, sliced into slivers
Fresh mint leaves, scissor-cut into slivers

Dressing

1 clove garlic, minced
1 T red wine vinegar
2 T olive oil

Pinch of salt
1 tsp turmeric

Peel the beet, cut into quarters and shred in the food processor. Combine dressing ingredients in a bowl and add shredded beets, sliced onion, and mint. Mix and serve on individual plates with a final grating of lemon zest. Serves two.

Simple Pear Salad with Balsamic Vinaigrette

1 whole fresh ripe pear, peeled, seeded, and sliced into thin crescents
1 dozen toasted pecans
Zest of half a lemon

Dressing

1 T balsamic vinegar
2 T olive oil

1 tsp Dijon mustard
1 tsp chopped mint leaves

Whisk mustard into vinegar and while whisking add olive oil. Whisk in mint. Spoon a pool of vinaigrette onto salad plates. Add the pear slices. Grate lemon zest into the center of pear slices. Sprinkle the edges with crushed pecans. Serves two.

Spinach Salad

5 cups spinach leaves   1 T poppy seeds
5 large white mushrooms, washed and dried

Wash and dry spinach leaves. Wash, dry and slice mushrooms

Dressing

1 T red wine vinegar   Pinch of salt
2 T olive oil   Lemon zest
1 tsp sesame oil

In a large salad bowl, combine vinegar, olive oil, sesame oil, and salt. Whisk. Add washed and dried spinach, and top with sliced mushrooms and poppy seeds. Let stand. Just before serving, add lemon zest and toss. Serves two.

Carrot Salad

2 cups carrots, grated
1 T lemon juice, freshly squeezed
½ tsp turmeric
½ tsp fresh ginger root, minced
2 T olive oil
Dark Bibb lettuce leaves, or another dark leaf lettuce
2 T fresh blueberries

Shred carrots by hand or in food processor. Toss carrots with lemon juice, turmeric, ginger, and olive oil. Serve carrot salad on a leaf of lettuce and sprinkle with blueberries. Serves two.

Warm Broccoli-Cauliflower Salad

½ head cauliflower and equal amount of broccoli, trimmed and cut into flowerets

Dressing

2 T red wine vinegar	1 T turmeric
4 T olive oil	1 T fresh rosemary or 1 tsp dried
½ tsp salt	1 tsp cayenne red pepper
2 cloves garlic, minced	Cracked black pepper

Steam vegetables until barely tender, about 10 minutes. While vegetables are still warm, pour dressing over and toss to mix.

To prepare dressing: In a medium salad bowl, mix vinegar, oil, salt, red pepper, turmeric, garlic, and rosemary. Add vegetables and stir. Crack pepper over salad. Serve while still warm. Serves two to four.

Zesty Beet Salad

1 medium-sized beet or two small beets

There are two ways to cook the beet:

▶ Put beet in a pot and fill with water to cover. Boil 20–25 minutes, or until a sharp knife easily enters the beet.

▶ Heat oven to 425 degrees. Place beet in a baking dish with ¼-inch of water. Cover the dish with a lid or aluminum foil and bake approximately 40 minutes, or until knife inserts easily.

After either baking or boiling the beet, peel and quarter it, and add the dressing while the beet is still warm. Toss and salt to taste. Bake large beets 50–60 minutes; small ones 30–40 minutes.

Dressing for Zesty Beet Salad

1 T apple cider vinegar	½ tsp turmeric
2 T olive oil	½ tsp ginger root, chopped

½ tsp cinnamon
1 pinch of cloves

1 small clove of garlic, chopped

Combine all ingredients in a bowl and whisk to incorporate.

Green and Yellow Bean Salad

½ pound each of fresh green and yellow string beans
4 T Lemon/Onion/Caper/Walnut Garnish (Pantry, page 97)
2 T parsley, chopped

Pinch off the stem end of the beans. Bring to boil enough water to cover the beans. When water is boiling, add beans and cook for 5 minutes or until just barely tender. Immediately pour off water and thoroughly rinse with cold water to halt cooking and retain color. Drain beans and set aside until ready to dress.

Arrange a bouquet of beans on a white salad plate and top with a spoonful of lemon/onion/caper/walnut relish and then chopped parsley

---

French Salad Composé

This salad is an intentional composition designed according to each cooks' preference and placement of ingredients.

Use any fresh vegetables, the greener or darker, the better. The trick is to dress each vegetable individually.

Suggested ingredients for a colorful palette include:

1 cup carrots, shredded, tossed with a little lemon juice and olive oil
1 cup fresh, raw beets, shredded, mixed with fresh mint, chopped
1 potato, boiled, peeled, and cubed, and drizzled while still warm with simple
    vinaigrette (recipe follows)
A handful of green beans steamed or cooked *al dente* (just barely tender), then
    sprinkled with fresh tarragon and a little salt and olive oil
3 tomatoes, peeled and quartered, sprinkled with lemon juice and olive oil, salt,
    and cracked pepper, and scissor-cut fresh basil and lemon zest

Roasted Red Pepper strips (Pantry, page 94)

A small nest of Kalamata or Niçoise olives

Combination of lettuces, such as dark Bibb, baby arugula, and radicchio

¼ cup Lemon Mayonnaise (Pantry, page 98) as topping

Garnishes

2 T pine nuts, raw or lightly toasted   Lemon zest

Simple Vinaigrette (in which to marinate potatoes)

2 T red wine vinegar

4 T olive oil

1 T fresh tarragon leaves, or ½ tsp dried tarragon

1 T fresh marjoram leaves and buds, or 1 tsp dried

½ tsp salt

Pepper, freshly cracked

1 clove garlic, minced

Combine vinegar and oil. Add tarragon, marjoram, salt, pepper, and garlic. Whisk and pour over potatoes. Adjust salt and pepper to taste.

Arrange lettuces on individual plates and create your vegetable composition; top with pine nuts and lemon zest, and pass a bowl of lemon-mayonnaise.

You could make a bistro dinner of this salad by adding a serving of steamed, poached, or grilled salmon topped with aioli and a sprinkling of fresh dill or fennel leaves. Yum! Serves two.

Black Bean Salad

1 cup dried black beans, or one 15-ounce can

1 cup dried pinto beans, or one 15-ounce can

½ cup dried black-eye peas, or one-half 15-ounce can

If using dried beans: Soak beans overnight (black beans separately). Rinse and pour fresh water over beans to cover. Cook beans over medium heat until tender—approximately 40–50 minutes. You may need to add more water as they cook. While beans are softening, begin the dressing in a large salad bowl.

Dressing

2 T red wine vinegar

Juice of half a lemon

Juice of half a regular lime, or juice of three Key limes

Zest of a whole lemon

2 T sweet onion, chopped

1 tsp turmeric

1 tsp fresh ginger root, chopped

2 cloves garlic, finely chopped

¼ cup olive oil

½ cup cilantro or ½ cup flat parsley, chopped

Salt and freshly ground pepper to taste

Combine all ingredients except the cilantro. If using dried beans, drain and rinse when tender. If using canned beans, drain and rinse, then heat in microwave for 2–3 minutes or on the stove until thoroughly warmed, about 10 minutes. While beans are still warm, add them to the dressing. Add salt to taste and a few grinds of black pepper. Add cilantro and enjoy! If you have to refrigerate this salad, be sure to refresh it with a squirt of fresh lemon juice and more zest when you are ready to serve it.

Avocado Salad

One whole unpeeled avocado

Dark lettuce leaves

Clover or sunflower sprouts, or a few leaves of dark Bibb lettuce

4 T blender vinaigrette

Dressing (makes 1½ cup)

1 small chunk of sweet onion

¼ cup red wine vinegar

1 cup olive oil

1 tsp dry mustard

1 T fresh tarragon or 1 tsp dry (try other herbs, or combinations of herbs—
dill, mint, chervil, basil)
1 T fresh parsley
½ tsp salt

To make the dressing: Combine all ingredients, except oil, in the food processor or blender. Whirl until onion and herbs are incorporated. While motor is running, slowly add one-third of the olive oil. Stop. Restart and add another third cup in a slow stream. Stop. Restart and add final third. Dressing should be the consistency of light mayonnaise. Salt to taste. Dressing will store in a covered jar in the fridge for 2 days. If refrigerated, shake thoroughly before serving.

To prepare the salad: Cut avocado in half lengthwise. Remove pit and place avocado on bed of lettuce leaves and sprouts. Fill cavity with thick dressing and top with a leaf of tarragon.

For a complete lunch, add a side of Black Olive/Tomato Relish (Pantry, page 98) and warm Pita Bread (pages 123–125). Serves two.

Mother's Fruit Salad

This salad still brings me "home." On long, hot summer days, even if we weren't hungry, Mother lured us to the table with this sweet salad of comfort and its surprising dressing.

1 whole pink grapefruit, peeled and sectioned
1 whole avocado, peeled and cut into thin slices
2 whole oranges, peeled and sectioned
1 banana, cut in diagonal slices
1 cup papaya (optional, if in season), cut into chunks
Half a pineapple, peeled, cored, and cut into sections
One dozen fresh strawberries, if in season
1 cup blueberries, if in season
1 mango, peeled and chopped

Any other fresh, in-season fruits that seem compatible, such as cantaloupe or honeydew, or reconstituted dried sour cherries. Combine fruit in large bowl and make dressing.

Dressing

3 T red wine vinegar	¼ cup honey
1 tsp dry mustard	White onion, about 2 T
½ tsp cayenne pepper	2 T mint leaves
½ tsp turmeric	1 clove garlic
1 T celery seed	½ cup olive oil

Combine all ingredients except oil in food processor. Puree until onion is incorporated.

While motor is running, drizzle in olive oil in steady stream until dressing thickens.

Pour dressing over fruit and mix the salad gently, so the fragile fruits are not disturbed. Serves six.

Cannellini Bean Salad with Fresh Herbs

1 cup dried cannellini beans soaked overnight and boiled for 20 minutes,
  or
1 15-ounce can of cannellini beans, drained and heated in microwave for 1.5 minutes, or on medium heat on the stove for 5 minutes, or until beans are heated through.
2 T balsamic vinegar
1 T olive oil
1 clove garlic, chopped
Juice of half a lemon, about 1 T
Juice of half a lime, about 2 tsp
1 tsp ginger root, chopped
½ tsp lavender (optional)
2 T each fresh cilantro, Italian parsley, basil, scissor-cut

1 T fresh mint leaves, chopped
A little salt and 2 grinds of freshly cracked pepper

Drain beans. While still warm, add remaining ingredients. Stir, taste, and serve warm. You will create an irresistible balsamic-citrus sauce on your plate, so serve with crusty rustic Italian bread. Serves two.

Poor Man's Caviar

1 medium eggplant
1 medium sweet onion, chopped
3 medium tomatoes, peeled and chopped (Pantry, pages 93–94)
2 cloves of garlic, minced
¼ cup olive oil
Squeeze of lemon juice
2 T red wine vinegar
Salt and cracked pepper to taste

Cut the top off the eggplant and place whole unpeeled eggplant in a casserole with about 1 inch of water. Cook in microwave 8–10 minutes or until eggplant is soft and skin is wrinkled, or place in baking dish with 2 inches of water, cover with foil, and bake at 350 degrees for 45 minutes or until skin is wrinkled.

Let eggplant cool. Peel skin using a sharp knife and scrape remaining flesh from the skin. Discard skin. Chop eggplant coarsely. In a medium-sized bowl, add onion, tomatoes, and garlic to eggplant; stir to mix. Add vinegar, lemon juice, and olive oil; stir. Add salt and freshly cracked pepper to taste.

Serve as a savory garnish, salad, or use as dip with toasted French bread rounds or triangles of pita bread. Makes 3 cups.

Hummus with Turmeric and Mint

1 cup of dried garbanzo beans, soaked and cooked
   or
1 15-ounce can garbanzo beans drained

1 T sesame tahini

2 T fresh lemon juice

1 T fresh lime juice

1 T fresh parsley

1 T sweet onion

1 clove garlic

½ cup olive oil

1 T sesame oil

½ tsp salt

Heat the garbanzo beans on the stove or in the microwave until just warmed through.

Combine all ingredients, except oil and salt, in food processor and puree until incorporated. With the motor running, slowly drizzle in the oils. Salt to taste. Makes 2 cups.

Arugula Salad with Hazelnuts, Almonds, Cherries, and Blue Cheese

Arugula is available in two varieties, baby and mature. The mature leaves are darker green, spicier, and have more defined lobes; the baby greens are lighter, with softer edges and a milder taste. Arugula is popular for more than its taste; it's high in iron, calcium, and vitamins A and C. Arugula is also versatile. Try it in salads, as a sautéed side dish, or added to soups and other cooked preparations. Arugula also makes a good bed for marinated vegetables.

4 cups mature arugula

2 T red wine vinegar

1 T olive oil

1 T walnut oil

1 T Jalapeño jelly, medium hot

½ tsp salt

2 T blue cheese, crumbled

2 T hazelnuts, lightly toasted and finely chopped

2 T slivered almonds, toasted but not chopped

1 dozen fresh Rainier or red cherries, pitted and halved. If cherries are not in
season, use apple slices, pear slices, or dried sour cherries reconstituted in
boiling water. (Bring 1 cup of water to a boil. Pour over dried cherries and
let stand for 5 minutes. Drain water off and squeeze excess water from
cherries.)

Wash arugula and spin dry. In a medium-sized salad bowl, combine red
wine vinegar, olive oil, walnut oil, and salt. Mix in the pepper jelly using a fork
or small whisk, until jelly is incorporated into the vinegar and oil. Salt to taste.
Add arugula. Just before serving add the cheese, cherries (or other fruit), and
nuts. Toss. This salad is great served with a one-pan roasted dinner (pages
158–159). Makes two servings.

Asparagus Salad

My favorite memory of eating asparagus was Simca and Jean's anniversary,
which occurred during our stay at the Hotel d'Orfeuil when we attended the
spa together. Simca had specifically ordered white asparagus for the occasion.
It wasn't Chef Troisgros' simple preparation of the rare white asparagus that
impressed me; it was watching Simca demonstrate the proper protocol for eating cold asparagus—with her fingers. Simca's famous anniversary asparagus
was quickly cooked in boiling water, removed, rinsed in cold water, and served
chilled on a white dinner plate with lemon zest grated over a pool of freshly
prepared lemon/mayonnaise for dipping. It was a white-on-white masterpiece
of simplicity with a sparkle of gold.

White asparagus is expensive and hard to find, so we use green asparagus,
which is rich in vitamin C and potassium. You'll need: 20–25 spears of fresh
asparagus, washed with tough bottom ends snapped off. (It used to be trendy
to peel asparagus, and if you wind up with tough asparagus, you will have to

peel it or—worse—pitch it. But with fresh tender stalks, you should only have to snap the bottom for even cooking.)

In a big kettle, bring 4–5 cups of water to a boil. When water is boiling, add asparagus all at once. Boil for 5 minutes and quickly drain water off. Immediately run cold water over asparagus to halt the cooking. Serves two.

Dressing Options

Raspberry-Mustard Vinaigrette
1 T raspberry vinegar or red wine vinegar
A squeeze of lemon juice (about 1 tsp)
2 tsp Dijon grainy mustard
¼ cup olive oil
Pinch of salt
A sprinkling of fresh raspberries

Combine vinegar, lemon juice, and mustard in a medium bowl and whisk to incorporate. While whisking, add the olive oil in a constant drizzle until dressing is slightly thickened. Taste. Add salt if needed.

Place chilled asparagus in bundle on serving plate and pour dressing over. Top with fresh raspberries. Eat with your fingers.

Lemon-Mayonnaise (recipe Pantry, page 98) is another good sauce for asparagus.

Poached Salmon Salad
¾ pound fresh salmon filet—sockeye, king, or Copper River are wonderful if
    you can obtain them
1 T sesame oil
5 cups water (or enough to cover salmon for poaching)
2 T prepared Genmaicha tea blend (green tea blended with roasted rice) or
    other green tea

1 tsp dried lovage or a small branch fresh lovage—if not available, use 2 tsp
fresh thyme and celery leaves.

Lemon zest

Salad Bed, on which to present poached salmon
Kalamata or Niçoise olives

1 T capers

2 medium fresh tomatoes, peeled (instructions Pantry, pages 93–94) and cut in
wedges

Half a Roasted Red Pepper, cut into long strips (Pantry, page 94)

½ fresh avocado, cut into thin slices

1 recipe of Lemon Mayonnaise (recipe Pantry, page 98)

1 recipe for simple vinaigrette (recipe below)

Half a head of dark Bibb lettuce or other dark lettuce, washed and spun dry.

1 T fresh dill, chopped

Dressing

1 T red wine vinegar   Pinch of salt

2 T olive oil

Combine salad ingredients in medium-sized bowl. Add washed and spun
lettuce and let stand. Drizzle with dressing and toss when ready to serve.

To poach the salmon: Bring water to a boil in heavy-bottomed skillet or
poaching pan. Add lovage or celery leaves and thyme, green tea—leaves and
all—and salmon. Poach over medium heat for 5–6 minutes. Remove from heat
but leave salmon in poaching water. Grate lemon zest over salmon and cover
with sesame oil. Cover pan. Let salmon rest off the heat for 5 minutes while
you prepare other ingredients.

Arrange lettuce on plates. Divide salmon filet into two portions. Add olives,
tomato wedges, and avocado slices around salmon. Pour Lemon Mayonnaise
over salad ingredients. Garnish with capers and chopped fresh dill. Serves two.

Warm Tilapia Salad

You'll need a steamer for this one. Tilapia is a delicate, subtly sweet white fish and deserves an equally respectful preparation so that you can taste the fish.

1 filet fresh tilapia, about 6 ounces

2 branches fresh thyme or ½ tsp dried thyme

1 squeeze of fresh lemon (preferably Meyer lemon)

Dressing

3 sweet white onion, sliced thinner than paper

1 T lemon juice

3 T olive oil

Salt and cracked pepper to taste

1 T capers or nasturtium buds

¼ of a roasted red pepper, cut julienne style

4 leaves red Bibb lettuce or dark lettuce, washed and gently torn to bite-size

Cilantro (or flat parsley)

Lemon zest

Steam tilapia with thyme and one squeeze of lemon juice, for about 5 minutes or until just flaky. Meanwhile, in a medium bowl, combine the onion slices, lemon juice, olive oil, capers, and salt. Reserve 1 T of dressing for bed of lettuce. Transfer tilapia from the steamer into the dressing. Add strips of roasted red pepper and gently flake the filet. Add salt and a small bit of cracked pepper to taste.

Serve on a bed of lettuce, dressed with reserved olive oil/lemon juice. Garnish with a few leaves of cilantro and one grating of lemon zest. Enjoy the salad while it is still warm. Serves two.

Endive Salad with Roasted Vegetables

Choose light-colored endive, with crisp leaves and a solid head.

One head of endive
12 stalks fresh asparagus, bottoms snapped off
Combination of mushrooms—shitake, portabello, large button
One medium red onion, quartered
2 T canola oil

Preheat oven to 400 degrees. Quarter button and shitake mushroom, and slice portabellos into ½-inch slices. On a 12-inch pizza pan or baking dish with edges, arrange mushrooms, asparagus, and red onion chunks. Drizzle canola oil over. Roast for 12–15 minutes. Wash endive leaves and spin dry.

Vinaigrette

1 T red wine vinegar   Pinch of salt
2 T olive oil   4 grinds of cracked black pepper

Whisk ingredients until oil and vinegar are incorporated. Remove vegetables from oven and arrange on a serving plate. While still warm, pour dressing over and serve. Serves two.

Beneficial Grains

There are many nutritional grains to explore from couscous and Quinoa to polenta and soba noodles in additional to the traditional pastas and rice.

Israeli Couscous with Vegetables

Serve with smoke-cooked salmon (pages 104–105) and peach salsa (see recipe for Mango Salsa, pages 104–105). If you can't find Israeli couscous, use the traditional smaller grain couscous or quinoa, but pursue the Israeli version. I found it in bulk at our local food co-op.

1 cup couscous	1 cup Olive Tower (Pantry, pages 96–97)
3 cups water	1 T pine nuts
1 cube chicken bouillon	1 T fresh blueberries
2 tsp turmeric	

In a medium saucepan, add 1 cup of couscous to 3 cups of water. Add chicken bouillon cube and turmeric. Simmer over medium heat until water is absorbed, about 15 minutes. Turn off heat, cover pan and let rest. Just before serving, fluff couscous with a fork and add Olive Tower, pine nuts, and fresh blueberries. Serves two.

Polenta with Roasted Vegetables and Steamed Tilapia

2½-inch rounds of precooked polenta (I use organic, fat-free, basil-garlic roll
of polenta from Quinoa Corp., which is available in many grocery stores
and food co-ops.)

1 medium Walla-Walla or other sweet onion, sliced in half straight across

2 medium sweet tomatoes, tops cut off

1 medium zucchini, cut in half lengthwise

1 whole garlic bulb with the very top cut off

2 T canola oil

Salt and freshly cracked pepper

½ roasted red pepper, cut in thin strips (instructions Pantry, page 94)

2 tilapia filets

1 T fresh lemon juice

A few pinches of dried thyme or 2 branches of fresh

2 shitake mushrooms, cut into thin strips

Preheat oven to 400 degrees. Drizzle 2 T canola oil on a pizza pan or oven-proof baking dish with an edge of at least ½ inch. Arrange in the pan the halved onion, cut side up, halved zucchini cut side down, tomatoes cut side up, and halved garlic bulb cut side up. Drizzle a bit of olive oil over onions, garlic, and tomatoes, and sprinkle with black pepper. Roast vegetables for 20 minutes. Add rounds of polenta to pan and continue roasting for another 10 minutes or until onions are golden.

Meanwhile, set up steamer for the tilapia. Sprinkle fish with a little salt, thyme, lemon juice, and thin strips of shitake mushrooms. Steam about 7–8 minutes or until fish is just flaky.

Arrange roasted vegetables and polenta on plates. Add a pool, about ¼ cup, of roasted red pepper sauce. Place tilapia with mushrooms in the pool. Top with a few leaves of cilantro and lemon zest. Serves two.

Quinoa Salad with Turmeric

Quinoa (keen-wah) is a popular, affordable, and widely available whole grain. It is gluten-free and an excellent source of protein (6 grams per serving).

½ cup quinoa, organic if available   1½ cups water

Salad

2 green onions, chopped

1 roasted red pepper, chopped (instructions Pantry, page 94)

1 clove garlic, chopped

1 tomato, chopped

Fresh chopped herbs: flat parsley, basil, dill, or mint, or a combination of fresh herbs

Dressing

1 T red wine vinegar   2 T olive oil

1 T balsamic vinegar   ½ tsp turmeric

A hearty squeeze of lemon   Salt and cracked pepper to taste

Combine quinoa with water and simmer for 15 minutes until tender and water is absorbed. Cover and let rest while you prepare dressing.

To make the dressing, in a salad bowl, combine vinegars, lemon juice, olive oil, garlic, turmeric, salt and pepper. Mix. Add warm quinoa and stir to coat. Salt and pepper to taste. Just before serving add roasted red pepper, chopped tomato, green onions, and herbs.

To make this an entire meal, add slices of delicate smoked chicken breast (recipe on pages 161–162). Serves two.

Mushroom Medley with Pasta

I used to make this with enoki mushrooms, but they are difficult for Mike to chew and swallow.

2 cups penne pasta

3 cups fresh mushrooms (Any combination of shitake, white button, oyster, chanterelles, or morels will do.)

2 tsp mushroom bouillon or 1 cube of chicken bouillon

1 cup water

½ tsp fresh nutmeg, grated

1 T fresh tarragon or ½ tsp dried tarragon

2 T sweet onion, finely chopped

1 tsp fresh lemon juice (Meyer lemon, if in season)

1 clove garlic, chopped

3 T Black Olive/Tomato Relish (Pantry, page 98)

2 T flat parsley, chopped

2 T olive oil

Clean mushrooms; cut bottom off oyster mushrooms and break into separate pieces. Slice other mushrooms.

Cook the pasta until tender, according to package directions. Drain and rinse in a colander. Let rest in colander until ready to serve.

In a large heavy skillet, combine water and bouillon, onion, garlic, and tarragon if using dried. If using fresh tarragon, wait and add it later. Bring bouillon mixture to a boil and add mushrooms. Stir, cooking mushrooms until they are tender and liquid is absorbed. Add nutmeg, fresh tarragon, and lemon juice. Stir. Add salt and freshly cracked pepper to taste.

Refresh the pasta by pouring boiling water over noodles in the colander.

Transfer noodles to large bowl and dress with 2 T olive oil and a little salt and cracked pepper to taste. Transfer warm noodles to serving platter and spoon mushroom medley over pasta. Top noodles with dollops of olive relish, and sprinkle parsley over all. Serves two.

Pasta with Eggplant and Red Sauce

2 cups fettuccine noodles

1 medium eggplant

3 cups Tomato Base (Pantry, page 96)

½ cup olive oil

1 T each of two or more fresh herbs: marjoram, parsley, thyme, oregano

One recipe of Pesto (Pantry, page 98)

Cook noodles in boiling water until tender. Drain and rinse in a colander. Set aside to reheat later.

Do not peel the eggplant. Cut it in half lengthwise, then cut into 1-inch chunks and put in a bowl. Sprinkle with salt and let stand for an hour to release some of the moisture. Rinse the eggplant and pat dry with paper towel.

In a heavy skillet, heat half the olive oil and add the eggplant. Stir to coat eggplant. Cook on medium heat until soft, stirring occasionally and adding more oil as needed. Add Tomato Base and fresh herbs and heat. Salt and pepper to taste.

To reheat pasta, bring 4 cups of water to boil and pour over pasta in a colander, then toss drained pasta with 2 T olive oil. Transfer pasta to a large bowl and mix with the eggplant and Tomato Base. Pour out onto serving platter. Top with pesto and pass extra at the table. Serves two.

Yamagata Soba Bowl

I've spent a lot of time in Yamagata—the Cherry Blossom capital of the world—visiting my Japanese friends, Ryodo and Miyoshi Ogata. Five years after Mike was diagnosed with Parkinson's, Ryodo invited Mike to serve as Visiting Scholar at Tohoku University of Arts and Design in Yamagata. For the month of January, we lived in a small apartment in Yamagata and experimented with local groceries on a two-burner stove.

The famous soba shops in Yamagata traditionally serve these buckwheat noodles in only their cooking liquid, which is said to be "good for the gut." I believe this is true, but we try to include a variety of soba-compatible ingredients in a one bowl, whole meal, layered presentation.

6–8 ounces soba noodles
½ cup carrots, grated
2 T nori (seaweed flakes)
4–5 shitake mushrooms, sliced
½ cup mushroom or vegetable stock
1 tsp sesame seeds
1 cup broccoli flowers precooked to just tender, drained and rinsed under cold
    water
1 cup precooked salmon (optional)

Bring 4 cups of water to a boil and add noodles. Boil for 5–7 minutes. Drain and rinse.

Toss noodles with nori (seaweed) flakes and sesame seeds.

Sauce for two bowls

4 T Kikkoman Tempura Dipping Sauce
1 T rice wine vinegar
1 tsp sesame oil
Juice of half a lemon

2 T cilantro, chopped
1 T fresh ginger, chopped
1 clove garlic, minced

Combine all sauce ingredients in a bowl, then divide sauce into two big soup bowls. Add vegetables and salmon to the sauce, then top with hot (drained) noodles and a grating of lemon rind. Serve with chopsticks, and be sure to tell guests that the sauce is in the bottom.

Try different ingredients. Some other good additions would be roasted, raw, or steamed asparagus; raw spinach or arugula; steamed or sautéed zucchini; or sliced raw button mushrooms. Serves two.

Soba Bowl Variation

This variation uses different vegetables, but the same sauce as the Yamagata Soba Bowl on pages 149–150.

Cooked soba noodles, drained
1 T olive oil
Half an avocado, cut into slices
1 Japanese eggplant, unpeeled and sliced at an angle ½-inch thick
1 Roasted Red Pepper (Pantry, page 94), cleaned and cut into long strips
Lemon zest
Green onion, chopped

Cover bottom of baking pan with olive oil. Place slices of eggplant in the pan. Roast for 15 minutes at 450 degrees.

Pour sauce into bottom of bowl and arrange eggplant slices around edge. Add cooked soba noodles, sliced avocado, and red pepper strips. Top with chopped green onion and lemon zest. Serves two.

Warm Sweet Brown Rice

Sweet brown rice is a whole grain—not processed like other rice; it only has the husk removed.

½ cup sweet brown rice
2½ cups water
1 T green onions, chopped

1 T flat parsley, chopped
2 medium tomatoes, chopped
½ avocado, chopped

Dressing
1 T red wine vinegar
1 T balsamic vinegar
2 T olive oil

½ tsp salt
1 clove garlic, chopped
Fresh tarragon

Add rice to water and bring to a boil. Reduce heat to simmer. Cover with a tight lid and cook for 40–50 minutes or until water is absorbed. Remove from heat and let cool until just warm. Add green onions, parsley, tomatoes, and avocado to the warm rice. To make dressing, combine ingredients in a bowl and whisk to incorporate. Pour dressing over rice and toss gently. Serve with a savory roasted free-range chicken. Makes two servings of rice.

Pizza Crust and Toppings

Crust

1½ cups warm water	1½ cups flour
1 T dry yeast	Pinch of salt
2 T olive oil	1 T olive oil for the pan

Add yeast to water and let stand until bubbly. Add 1 T of the olive oil and pinch of salt. Stir in 1 cup of flour and mix until smooth. Cover with clean towel and let stand in warm place until doubled, about 20 minutes. Add remaining 1 T olive oil to dough and mix. Sprinkle remaining ½ cup flour on a good kneading surface and knead into the dough until smooth. Let rest another 20 minutes. (At this point you can punch dough down and store in a zipper-close plastic bag for up to 24 hours. When working with refrigerated dough, let it rest in a warm place for 15 minutes before shaping it.)

Preheat oven to 350 degrees. Prepare a pizza pan by drizzling 2 T olive oil on surface. Drop pizza dough in center of pan and work dough gently out to the edges. Let rest about 10 minutes before topping. Or, shape individual pizzas on a baking sheet.

Simple Topping

Half a medium sweet onion, sliced into paper-thin rounds
2 medium tomatoes, cut into thin slices
2 large cloves garlic, chopped
Rosemary 1 tsp dried or 2 T fresh
1 tsp dried basil
2 tsp oregano
Pepper, freshly cracked

1 tsp sea salt (try a flavored one, such as merlot!)

Spread onion slices over pizza dough. Place tomato slices around the edges. Sprinkle with herbs, salt and garlic. Crack pepper over the top. Let rest in a warm place for about 10 minutes before baking.

Bake about 40 minutes or until crust is golden brown. Remove from oven, and while still warm, drizzle one or two T of olive oil over the top.

If you have fresh basil, scissor-cut it over the top after baking. Makes one 12-inch round pizza crust or four individual pizzas. Partner this with a great salad from those on pages 128 to 144, and you have a complete dinner!

Another Good Pizza Topping

4–6 canned anchovies   2 cups Tomato Base (Pantry, page 96)

Prepare pizza dough as above. Spread with Tomato Base. Drizzle a little (1 T) olive oil on top of tomato sauce. Arrange anchovies on top of tomato sauce. Let rest 10 minutes. Bake 40 minutes, until golden brown.

Cracked Wheat Bread

If you do not want to make bread, of course you can use any bread but I recommend a whole-grain bread for the most benefit. You can make this in a bread machine or by hand. This makes two long loaves.

2 cups boiling water
2 cups cracked wheat
1 T dry yeast
½ cup warm water
¾ cup honey
2 T butter substitute (Earth Balance or Smart Balance)
1 T salt
4–4½ cups white unbleached flour
1 T yellow cornmeal
1 whole egg

In a large mixing bowl, combine boiling water with cracked wheat. Dissolve yeast in ½ cup warm water. When the cracked wheat is cooled to warm add yeast mixture, honey, and butter. Stir and add 2 cups of flour. Mix well. Then add 2 more cups of flour and stir to incorporate. Let dough rest 10 minutes.

Sprinkle remaining ½ cup of flour on a kneading surface and knead dough for about 15 minutes until all flour is incorporated and dough is elastic but still a little sticky. Cover dough with a towel and let rise until double, about 1 hour. Punch dough down and shape into two balls. Let rest 10 minutes.

Alternatively, a bread machine can be used to knead the dough.

Preheat oven to 350 degrees. Form each ball into 15 × 8-inch rectangles and roll, jelly-roll style, into logs, pinching the seams together with your fingers. Place each loaf, seam down, on a baking sheet that has been sprinkled with 1 T yellow corn meal. Wash the tops of loaves with one whole egg lightly whipped with a fork. Using a sharp knife, slash tops of the loaves diagonally. Cover with a towel and let rise in a warm place for half an hour.

Bake bread 45 minutes or until golden brown. When it's done, it should sound hollow when tapped on top. Let cool a few minutes before slicing.

Quinoa and Israeli Couscous

This makes an excellent warm bed for a salmon fillet poached in green tea! (Recipe for poached salmon, pages 141–142.)

½ cup quinoa	1 T fresh lemon juice
½ cup Israeli couscous	2 tsp fresh lime juice
3 cups water	2 T green onion, chopped
2 tsp mushroom bouillon	1 medium tomato, chopped
½ tsp cinnamon	2 T olive oil
Scraping of nutmeg	Pinch of salt and cracked pepper
1 tsp turmeric	2 large leaves of dark lettuce

Bring water to a boil, add bouillon, couscous, and quinoa. Cook over medium heat for about 20 minutes until grains are tender and water is absorbed. Remove from heat. Add cinnamon, nutmeg, turmeric, lemon juice, and lime juice; mix. Add olive oil and stir. Salt to taste. Serve warm on leaves of dark lettuce. Serves two.

Vegetables

Mashed potatoes with an antioxidant twist, a one pan roasted meal, asparagus and sweet potato delight.

Mashed Potatoes with Turmeric

3 medium potatoes (I like Yukon Gold potatoes when in season. They're sweeter and deeper in color than white potatoes.)

2 tsp turmeric

1 T butter substitute (Earth Balance or Smart Balance)

4 T plain soy or almond milk

½ cup Black Olive Tower (Pantry, pages 96–97)

2 T pine nuts

Peel and quarter three medium potatoes. Cover with water and boil until tender. Pour off water. Mash potatoes with turmeric and butter substitute and soy or almond milk until smooth.

Top each serving with ¼ cup of Black Olive Tower mixture, then sprinkle with pine nuts—toasted or raw.

Another fun idea for mashed potatoes is to stir a handful of dried sour cherries into warm potatoes *after* mashing.

Also, try substituting rutabagas for potatoes. Just peel and cut up like a potato, then boil in water until tender. Transfer cooked rutabagas to the food processor, add 2 T butter substitute, and whirl until smooth. Stir in reconstituted dried sour cherries. Salt to taste. It's really lovely! Serves two.

Asparagus with Diced Tomatoes

16–20 stems of fresh, young, sturdy asparagus
2 medium ripe tomatoes peeled (Pantry, pages 93–94)
1 T canola oil
1 T olive oil
1 T fresh basil, chopped
Lemon zest

We're going to cook this asparagus twice, but lightly both times. First, bring water to boil while snapping the tough ends off asparagus. Once the water is boiling, drop asparagus in and cook for about 4 minutes. Immediately pour off water and rinse asparagus thoroughly with cold water to halt the cooking. Drain asparagus and let dry on paper towel. Better yet, if you have a steamer, use it to just barely cook the asparagus.

Chop tomatoes and sprinkle with lemon zest, olive oil, and fresh basil.

Add canola oil to a heavy-bottomed skillet and heat. Add steamed or boiled asparagus and toss until coated. Arrange asparagus on each plate, top with chopped tomatoes. Add a grind of sea salt and cracked pepper to taste. Serves two.

Sweet Potato Rounds with Smoky Sea Salt

1 whole unpeeled deep orange sweet potato (yam)
2 T olive oil
Smoky or plain sea salt

Preheat oven to 375 degrees.

Wash sweet potato and cut into ½-inch round slices. Drizzle a baking pan with olive oil and place sweet potato slices in pan. Bake in oven 20–25 minutes. Drain on paper towel. Sprinkle with sea salt. Serve warm. Makes two servings

---

Roasted Vegetables with (or without) Chicken Breast

You can do a lot with the concept of a one-pan roasted dinner. This combination is our absolute favorite. And, since Mike usually does the dishes, he loves the one-pan preparation! I like to roast or grill fish and chicken on a bed of herbs, usually lovage, arugula, sorrel, or parsley, and accompany them with this medley of roasted vegetables.

1 sweet potato, unpeeled, washed, and cut into 1-inch rounds

2 medium raw beets, peeled and cut in 1-inch rounds

1 medium sweet onion, cut in half

2 medium tomatoes, tops cut off

2 lemons, cut in 1-inch rounds, seeds removed (this is a good place for Meyer
  lemons if you have them, otherwise a sour lemon will work)

1 chicken breast on a bed of sorrel, lovage, arugula, or flat parsley

A pinch of dried lovage or marjoram

2 tsp smoky or plain sea salt

1 whole head of garlic, with the top cut off

2 T Balsamic vinegar

Olive oil

1 T fresh lime juice

Preheat oven to 400 degrees. Prick the surface of the halved onion with a sharp knife. Drizzle 1 T olive oil on a 12-inch pizza pan or an ovenproof baking dish. Place rounds of sweet potato, beets, the halved onion on a bed of sorrel, arugula or lovage on the baking dish add the head of garlic, cut side up, and chicken breast., Add tomatoes and lemon slice to the pan. Drizzle another 2 T olive oil over the vegetables.

Roast the vegetables and chicken for 30 minutes or until a sharp knife easily pierces the beets. Remove from oven and drizzle everything with balsamic vinegar. Remove the skin from chicken and sprinkle the chicken with marjoram, sea salt, and lime juice. Cut chicken breast in half.

Divide vegetables and chicken between two plates. Arrange lemons in the middle of the plate. Spoon or pour any cooking juices onto the lemon slices. Poke at the lemon slices while you eat to release even more juice! Serves two.

———————

Bahia de Kino Recipes

Two recipes that bring back the flavor and scents of Kino Bay, Mexico. I learned the taco-toasting technique from our Mexican neighbor, Lourdes Devaney.

Toasted Corn Tortilla with Salsa

4 6-inch corn tortillas
½ cup cooked and marinated potatoes (pages 133–134, French salad composé)
1 15-ounce can cannellini beans, drained and heated in microwave for 2 minutes
      or on the burner 5 minutes until heated through
1 T lemon juice, freshly squeezed
1 T olive oil
Pinch of salt
3 medium radishes, thinly sliced
½ avocado, thinly sliced
4 T salsa (recipe for homemade salsa follows)
4 key limes, cut in half
1 T cilantro, chopped

After heating the beans, add the lemon juice, olive oil, and salt. Let rest. Toast corn tortillas over the gas flame or directly on the coil burner until the edges are browned, flip the tortilla over—about 15 seconds per side.

Place tortillas on plates. Add potatoes and beans, top with avocado slices, radishes, salsa, and chopped cilantro. Serve with halved Key limes.

Chunky Salsa

1 jalapeño pepper, seeded and chopped

2 Anaheim peppers, seeded and chopped

1 Serrano pepper, seeded and chopped

1 T sweet white onion, chopped

1 clove of garlic, minced

¼ cup cilantro, chopped

3 medium tomatoes, chopped

½ tsp honey or agave syrup

1 T red wine vinegar

Juice from 4 Key limes

2 T olive oil

Stir ingredients together and you're done!

Smoke-Roasted Chicken

In my attempt to capture the essence of the iron wood fires of Old Kino, I made this chicken at our *casita* in Kino Bay on a small grill using big chunks of mesquite, and I started the fire with pecan wood kindling and a week's worth of newspaper. I used another piece of pecan for smoking. The whole process took almost all day. I'll never match the taste we experienced in Kino, but this recipe comes close to the memory.

1 whole 3-pound free-range or organic chicken

Salt

One whole orange or one pink grapefruit, peeled and cut into chunks

Smoking wood—apple, plum, alder, or pear

Rinse chicken inside and out with cold water. Dry with paper towels. Sprinkle salt inside cavity and fill with cut fruit. Let chicken rest while you start the fire.

Place a 5-inch chunk of smoking wood (or ¼ pound of chips) in water to soak for half an hour. Fill charcoal chimney to the top with charcoal, paper in the bottom (no lighter fluid), and light. When the coals are red, pour them out at one end of fire pit or grill. Add wet smoking-wood to coals. Replace cooking grill.

Place a heavy cookie sheet directly on the grill over the coals. Place chicken on grill beside the cookie sheet. *Close the lid* and cook for 1 hour. Check chicken and turn it around, but not over. Roast for another 45 minutes. The chicken cooks by radiant heat and is flavored by the smoking chips. The skin will turn a sumptuous amber color and the meat will be very juicy.

After the chicken is roasted, remove it from the grill. Let it rest for a few minutes. Remove skin and slice to suit recipe. This meat will last for 4–5 days in the refrigerator if it is well covered.

Serve with Chunky Salsa (page 161) and toasted corn tortillas.

If you don't have a grill, you can prepare a whole chicken the same way using smoky sea salt inside and out, and roasting the chicken in the oven at 400 degrees for 20 minutes per pound. Also, see the smoke-roasted chicken recipe on page 161. Serves six.

Breakfast Ideas

We're hearing a lot about eating non-traditional and nutrition-packed food for breakfast. For example at a recent Parkinson's wellness conference, a naturopath suggested eating butternut squash soup for breakfast. Open the "box" and try something new! Following are mildly altered traditional recipes and one "out of the box."

Eggs with Crab and Hollandaise

Our traditional Christmas breakfast has always been eggs Benedict with ham. Since moving to Bellingham, we've discovered the beauty of fresh Dungeness crab.

The Basics
English muffins
Meat from half a Dungeness crab or canned crab meat
2–4 eggs
2 medium tomatoes, tops cut off
1 T each fresh basil and tarragon
Salt and cracked pepper
8–10 Kalamata olives, chopped
1 recipe of hollandaise (below)

One-Egg Hollandaise Sauce
1 whole egg
2 T lemon juice
½ tsp cayenne pepper

Pinch of salt
¼ pound unsalted butter

In the food processor, combine egg, lemon juice, cayenne, and pinch of salt and puree for 30 seconds. Melt 8 T unsalted butter in microwave until almost boiling. With the motor running, pour hot butter into egg mixture in a slow stream until all butter is added. Let rest.

Assembly: Preheat oven to 375 degrees. Place a little butter in two custard dishes and put in oven to melt the butter. Remove from oven and add one egg to each dish. Return eggs to oven to bake until done—20 minutes.

Place tomatoes in custard dishes, sprinkle with chopped basil, tarragon, olive oil, salt and pepper, and bake in oven for 20 minutes.

Spread English muffins with a little butter and warm in the oven—don't toast, or they will be too hard to cut.

Combine crab flakes in a bowl with 1 tsp unsalted butter and heat in microwave about 2 minutes. Add 1 tsp lemon juice and mix into crab.

Arrange muffins on plates. Add egg and top with crab. Pour hollandaise over crab and top with chopped olives. Serve beside savory roasted tomato. Serves two.

If you're substituting a slice of roasted tomato for the fresh crab, leave out the whole baked tomatoes.

To roast tomato slices: Preheat oven to 450 degrees. Cut a medium tomato into 1-inch slices. Add 1 T olive oil to a shallow baking dish. Add tomato slices. Season with a little salt and pepper and roast for 5–7 minutes. Add chopped fresh basil or dried basil to tomatoes and continue assembly as directed above, using tomato instead of crab meat.

Everyday Cereal

Our favorite winter time breakfast is either oatmeal or malt-o-meal. What I like best is the opportunity to start the day with a vehicle for sour or tart dried cherries. After I stir the cereal into the boiling water, I turn the heat off, add a handful of cherries and another of raisins, cover the cereal pot, and let it rest while I make tea.

For breakfast in the warm months, Mike eats a bowl of whole grain cold cereal with an equal amount of fresh blueberries, blackberries, or raspberries.

Simple 30-Second Omelet

It was an early spring evening in Provence. The gardener was down the hill pruning the grape vines in the rain. Simca had been teaching all day, and her cook Jeanette was not feeling well.

"So, tonight," Simca announced to her husband, Jean, and me, "we will enjoy a simple parsley omelet with a glass of Beaujolais by the fire."

The gardener delivered a bundle of grape vine clippings to the door and Jean started a fire from that bounty. Simca and I hustled to the kitchen where, for the first time, I had the opportunity to observe the Master cooking in her *own* kitchen. Omelets are always good for breakfast, but sometimes Mike and I give ourselves permission to enjoy a simple omelet by the fire on a rainy Sunday night.

4 eggs

A pinch of salt

A couple grinds of cracked pepper

1 T unsalted butter

4 T parsley, chopped

1 T fresh tarragon leaves

Extra tarragon and parsley for garnish

In a medium bowl, using a fork whip 4 eggs together with half the parsley and half the tarragon, and salt and pepper to taste.

Heat a 7-inch omelet pan or heavy skillet on high heat with the butter. Tilt the pan to distribute the butter over bottom of the pan. When the foam has subsided, the pan is hot.

Pour the eggs into the pan. Begin sliding the pan back and forth vigorously, moving the egg mass over the bottom of the pan. Sprinkle the eggs with remainder of herbs. Using the fork as an aid, begin lifting the edge closest to you, gently folding it toward the opposite side. With the serving plate at your side, tilt the pan and fold the omelet over itself onto a plate. Divide omelet in two and sprinkle extra herbs over the top. Serves two.

Yamagata Breakfast Rice Bowl with Salmon

In 1995, Ryodo and Miyoshi visited us in Northfield, bringing gifts, including a few packages of dried breakfast food. I prepared the food immediately.

The ingredients were freeze-dried rice and salmon flakes, sesame seeds, seaweed (nori), and other seasonings. The cooking instructions were simple: place contents of envelope in 1 cup water and microwave for 2 minutes. It was delicious.

When I had used up our gift, I asked Ryodo if he would send more. His response was swift, saying each small packet cost $10, plus shipping. Then he told me how to make my own! This recipe is a satisfactory facsimile:

¼ cup precooked salmon
½ cup precooked sticky rice (be sure to wash your rice twice before cooking.)
2 T nori flakes
1 tsp sesame seeds
1 tsp sweet onion, shredded
Pinch of sea salt
1 tsp sesame oil
A pinch of cayenne pepper or pinch of Thai chili pepper
Juice of half a Key lime
1 T cilantro, chopped

Combine all ingredients except sesame oil, lime, and cilantro. Heat the rice for 2 minutes in microwave. Add sesame oil, lime juice, and cilantro, and then stir to mix. Serves two.

Desserts

Warm Fruit Compote

4 whole plums, pitted and halved

½ cup dried apricots

1 dozen dried sour cherries

1 whole fresh pear, peeled, seeded, and quartered

1 tsp ginger root, chopped

½ tsp cinnamon

1 fresh mango, peeled and cut into bite-sized pieces

1½ cup port wine

¼ cup agave syrup or ½ tsp powdered or liquid stevia

4 dollops plain soy yogurt

1 cinnamon stick per serving

Pour the port and agave syrup into a medium-sized saucepan. Add apricots, dried cherries, ginger, and cinnamon. Bring liquid to a boil and reduce heat to simmer. Add remainder of the fruit and continue poaching on low heat for 10 minutes. Remove fruit with a slotted spoon and reduce sauce to the consistency of syrup. Arrange fruit in serving dishes and pour a little sauce over it, topping each serving with a dollop of plain soy yogurt and a stick of cinnamon.

Note: If you have access to rose geranium flowers or leaves, add several leaves to the port for poaching. Remove the geranium leaves before serving. Top the compote with one flower of the rose geranium. Serves four.

——————

Blueberry Tart

Tart Shell

3 T unrefined sugar

2 cups mixed finely ground nuts—walnuts, pecans, hazelnuts

3 T softened unsalted butter

Zest of half a lemon

½ tsp cinnamon

Preheat oven to 350 degrees. Chop nuts with sugar, lemon zest, cinnamon, and butter in a food processor until moderately fine. Press nut mixture into 8-inch pie pan and bake for 15 minutes or until golden brown. Cool the shell.

Filling

3 cups fresh blueberries or a combination of blueberries and blackberries

½ cup blackberry or currant jelly

2 T cassis (black currant liquor)

2 gratings of nutmeg

1 grating of lemon zest

1 grating of orange zest

Rose geranium leaves (optional)

Add fresh berries to the baked and cooled shell. Spoon jelly into a bowl and melt it in microwave about 1 minute or until it's completely liquid. (Or, heat jelly over low heat in a pan on the stove.) Then, quickly add cassis, lemon and orange zest, a grating of nutmeg, and the rose geranium leaves to the jelly. Mix together, remove the leaves, then pour jelly over the blueberries.

In late summer and early fall, I top each serving with a beautiful pink, aromatic edible flower from the rose geranium plant outside my kitchen window. What a sight, what a smell, what a taste! Almost any geranium flower will work to decorate each slice. Serves six.

Mango-Pineapple-Strawberry Ice

2 cups fresh pineapple chunks

2 cups mango, chopped

½ cup strawberries

½ cup water

¼ cup honey

1 T lemon juice

3 T agave syrup or a drop of stevia

In a food processor, blend pineapple, mango, strawberries, water, agave syrup (or stevia), honey, and lemon juice until smooth. Pour into a 9-inch-square pan and freeze for 2 hours, or until firm. Cut the mixture into cubes. Place in a food processor and blend until smooth. Pack in airtight freezer container and freeze until use. Can be frozen up to a month.

To serve: Scoop fruit ice into glass dish and arrange fresh cut fruit around the edges. Top with zest of lemon and orange. Serves four.

Chocolate Torte

This dark chocolate cake is moist and rich. You'll only want to eat a small slice, so you'll have plenty to save for another meal.

The Cake

4 T softened unsalted butter

4 ounces bittersweet dark chocolate chips, preferably 60 percent cacao

2 eggs separated

1/3 cup sugar

1 tsp pure vanilla

¾ cup flour

Pinch of salt

½ cup water

Preheat oven to 350 degrees. In microwave or double-boiler, melt butter with 4 ounces of chocolate (about 1.5 minutes in microwave). Let cool until just warm. Then combine all ingredients except the flour and egg whites in a mixing bowl and beat until incorporated. Fold in the flour. Beat egg whites to soft peaks and fold into batter. Pour batter into an 8-inch spring-form cake pan and bake 30 minutes. Remove cake from pan and let cool. Glaze with chocolate.

Glaze
4 ounces softened unsalted butter
4 ounces dark bittersweet high-cacao chocolate chips, 60 percent cacao
½ cup slivered almonds
Fresh fruit

Spread the almonds on a cookie sheet and toast in 350-degree oven about 10 minutes or until just turning golden. Remove and cool.

In microwave or double boiler, melt butter and chocolate together until soft (about 1.5 minutes in microwave). Mix butter and chocolate together with a fork and let stand until just warm.

Stir toasted almonds into chocolate-butter mixture and frost the cake. Serve with a colorful variety of fresh fruit—sliced strawberries, fresh raspberries, sliced kiwi, fresh cherries, currants, or blackberries.

Treats and Snacks

Chocolate Almond Candies to Serve with Fruit

8 ounces dark chocolate with high cacao content

½ cup slivered almonds

2 T powdered unsweetened chocolate

In a 400-degree oven, toast slivered blanched almonds until just barely golden, about 10 minutes. Cool and crush into small pieces.

In a medium bowl, melt dark chocolate with high cocoa content (such as Ghirardelli 60 percent cocoa) in double-boiler, or 1½ minutes in microwave.

Using a fork, quickly whisk almonds into melted chocolate and pour onto waxed paper to cool.

When cooled enough to handle, shape chocolate into 12 round balls and roll in powdered unsweetened chocolate. Serve immediately, or store in tightly covered container in the refrigerator. These are wonderful when served with red grapes or cherries.

Antioxidant Smoothie Lollapalooza

This is for that middle-of-the-night sweets "fix." Mike wakes up at night and usually likes a piece of toast with honey accompanied by an already prepared smoothie waiting for him in the fridge.

1 banana
½ cup frozen blackberries
½ cup frozen blueberries
½ tsp cinnamon
2 slices fresh ginger root
A tiny pinch of cloves
Two scrapings of nutmeg
Dash of cardamom
½ cup tart cherry juice or other antioxidant fruit drink
6 ounces of plain soy yogurt or cultured coconut milk
3–4 leaves of fresh mint

Combine all ingredients (except cherry juice) in food processor and puree to incorporate the banana. When contents are smooth, with motor running, add cherry juice. Too thick? Add more juice.

If you want to serve this for a dessert, pour it into tall glasses and top with fresh berries, a sprig of mint, a flower of rose geranium, or a flower of bee borage. Serves 2.

Mixed Nuts with Raisins and Dried Sour Cherries

Nothing is easier or more nutritious than this snack. I've discovered that if I prepare a combination of healthy nuts and leave them sitting around alluringly in a pottery bowl on the counter, they disappear. The sweetness of these nuts is enhanced by toasting. You'll be surprised!

½ cup slivered almonds

½ cup walnuts

½ cup hazelnuts

¼ cup raisins

½ cup pecans

½ cup dried sour cherries

Preheat oven to 350 degrees. On a cookie sheet, combine the nuts. Toast in oven for 15 minutes or until the almonds are lightly golden. Then mix the dried fruit with the nuts.

Edamame Beans: Another Good Antioxidant Snack

I love edamame (soy beans) and, for ease of preparation, you can find already shelled edamame beans in the frozen food aisle. They are emerald green, crisp, and tasty!

Heat ¼ cup frozen edamame beans in microwave for 3 minutes, or steam them for 5 minutes. While they're warm, sprinkle with a little olive oil, fresh cracked pepper, and a tiny bit of sea salt. They are great for an afternoon snack with a cup of Genmaicha green tea to further enhance the flavor and enjoyment of the beans!

In Conclusion

Hopefully, this book has introduced you to a recipe, a new spice or herb, or another ingredient that surprised you. Maybe you learned something helpful from Carolyn Stinson's contributions or Nanette Davis' perspective on caregiving.

As you know from our story, in the beginning, Mike refused to exercise—he built and drove his cars, and he made his art.

Now, he goes to yoga twice a week, and he is still driving his old cars to town and walking a mile every day. Seventeen years ago, Mike's original dose of Sinemet® was three pills a day—today, he's increased his daily dose by one and a half pills. He is 77 years old, and this year we'll celebrate our 30th wedding anniversary. Mike's comment: "I'd love another 30 years. I'd like it better without PD. But most people make it easier to have a good life. I get assistance and encouragement every day, and I've had a lot more opportunity to educate people about PD."

Mike is still making his art. He works on sketches for new yard sculptures, 7-foot-tall stainless steel "tubes of light" with soaring bird images laser-cut in a random design around the structures to allow the light to shine through.

If you ever feel like Mike does when he struggles to button his shirt, *like you're trying to build a Model T with a sled*, and things are just discouraging and overwhelming, try to remember that you *do* have some control. You *can do something*! Every day, three times a day (or more), you can feed your brain what it craves for optimal health. You have to eat, so why not eat food that works *for* you—not against you?

The science of nutrition is dynamic, and our pantry expands accordingly, with more savory herbs and spices, fruits and vegetables. Just recently, I discovered a new herb, lime thyme!

I passionately believe that prevention is the most economically efficient cure for what ails us—socially and medically. With respect to proper diet as a preventative approach to better health, I am encouraged by the work of leaders such as Dr. Dean Ornish, who has scientifically proven that heart disease can indeed be reversed with lifestyle changes. I hope we all see the day when there's scientific proof that a lifestyle that includes proper nutrition and exercise has the power to slow the progression of Parkinson's disease, adding years of quality to your life.

Thank you for spending time with us in Northfield, Kino Bay, and in our Bellingham kitchen, dining room, pantry, and garden.

A final thought: If Mike can joyfully embrace exercise and yoga, and I can adapt to cooking with a minimum of butter and cream, anything is possible!

Bon Appetit!

Resources

GENERAL BOOKS ON PARKINSON'S DISEASE

A number of books specific to Parkinson's disease (PD) are available from Amazon and other online book seller sites. Search on the keywords "Parkinson's Disease." For books about exercises for people with PD, search on the keywords "Exercise + Parkinson's Disease."

Three books, two specifically dealing with life with PD and one dealing more generally with healthy aging and lifestyle are:

- ▶ *Parkinson's Disease: A Complete Guide for Patients and Families*, by William J. Weiner and Lisa Shulman (Johns Hopkins University Press, 2006).
- ▶ *Parkinson's Disease 300 Tips for Making Life Easier*, by Shelley Peterman Schwarz, (Demos Medical Publishing, 2006). Simple and important, time-saving tips for people with PD covering all your activities of daily living.
- ▶ *Living Agelessly: Creating a Lifestyle for Midlife and Beyond*, by Linda Altoonian (Diamedica Publishing, 2009).

ORGANIZATION WEBSITES

American Parkinson Disease Association
"Ease the burden and find a cure"
www.apdaparkinson.org
email: info@parkinsonsaction.org

Michael J. Fox Foundation for Parkinson's Research
www.michaeljfox.org

National Parkinson Foundation
"Knowledge is power and hope is everything"
www.parkinson.org

Northwest Parkinson's Foundation, Improving the Quality of Life
Seattle, Washington; publishes *The Parkinson's Post*
www.nwpf.org

Parkinson's Action Network (PAN)
The voice of Parkinson's on public policy issues
www.parkinsonsaction.org
email: info@parkinsonsaction.org

Parkinson's Disease Foundation (PDF)
Hope through research, education, and advocacy
www.pdf.org

Parkinson's Research Foundation
Current research, news, entertainment, and blog site. This site advertises the popular Parkinson's Cruise, designed specifically for the comfort and education of people with PD and their caregivers.
www.parkinsonsresearchfoundation.org

Diet, Health, Herbs, and Antioxidants

▶ The McCormick Science Institute, McCormick & Company, Inc. has an excellent website devoted to advancing the health benefits of spices and herbs: www.mccormickscienceinstitute.com

▶ To aid you in your search for current news and science relating to antioxidants: www.antioxidantshealth.org/

▶ For more antioxidant food sources: www.myclevelandclinic.org/heart/prevention

▶ *Anti-inflammatory Foods for Health: Hundreds of Ways to Incorporate Omega-3's Rich Foods into Your Diet to Fight Arthritis, Cancer, Heart Disease and More* by Barbara Rowe and Lisa Davis (Fairwinds Press, Lions Bay, Canada, 2008)

▶ *The Antioxidant Save-Your-Life Cookbook: 150 Nutritious High Fiber, Low-Fat Recipes to Protect Yourself Against the Damaging Effects of Free Radicals*, Jane Kinderlehrer and Daniel A. Kinderlehrer M.D. (Newmarket Press, New York, 2007).

▶ *The China Study: Startling Implications for Diet, Weight Loss and Long-Term Health*, by T. Colin Campbell, PhD and Thomas M. Campbell II (BenBella Books Dallas, Texas, 2006).

Exercise/Meditation

▶ Jay L. Alberts, Ph.D., of the Associate Staff, Department of Biomedical Engineering and Center for Neurological Restoration, Cleveland Clinic, Cleveland, Ohio, sponsors a website devoted to the benefits of exercise and meditation: http://www.lerner.ccf.org/bme/alberts/.

▶ The Transcendental Meditation® website outlines the health and quality-of-life benefits of meditation: www.tm.org

▶ Paul Lam's Tai Chi DVDs by Paul Lam include standard and disease-specific tai chi exercises. Available at www.amazon.com

▶ *Delay the Disease: Exercise and Parkinson's Disease*, by David Zid (Columbus Health Works Productions, 2007). Author Zid, a professional fitness instructor, takes PD readers through a well-photographed, step-by-step exercise program specifically designed for people with Parkinson's.

SPIRITUALITY AND EMPOWERMENT

▶ *The Biology of Belief: Unleashing the Power of Consciousness, Matter, & Miracles* by Bruce Lipton, Ph.D. Lipton, a scientist and philosopher, demonstrates from a scientific viewpoint that our lifestyle is in control of our health. This fascinating and courageous contribution will empower readers to engage and take charge of their lives. (Mountain of Love/Elite Books, Santa Rosa, CA, 2005; www.BruceLipton.com).

▶ *The Divine Matrix: Bridging Time, Space, Miracles, and Belief* by Gregg Braden. (Hay House: Carlsbad, California, 2008).

CAREGIVING

▶ *Blessed Is She: Women's Stories of Choice, Challenge and Commitment* by Nanette J. Davis, Ph.D. (House of Harmony Press, 2008).

▶ *Caregiving: The Spiritual Journey of Love, Loss, and Renewal*, Beth Witrogen McLeod. An extraordinary presentation of the challenges and rewards of caregiving including McLeod's own spiritual journey through the pain and growth of caring for her parents. (John Wiley & Sons, Inc. 1999).

▶ *The Comfort of Home: A Complete Guide for Caregivers 3rd Edition*, Maria M. Meyer with Paula Derr, RN. (Care Trust Publications LLC, 2007).

GROCERY INFORMATION

▶ Earth Balance (non-dairy butter substitute), ALA Omega-3: 400 mg per serving, 25% DV. Paramus, NJ 07652-1432. Phone 201-568-9300: www.earthbalancenatural.com

▶ Support your local farmer's market; find what's ripe and ready nearest you: www.localharvest.org

▶ The Spice House, Chicago. Spices, herbs, salts, seasonings, extracts, and organic versions of many items: www.thespicehouse.com

▶ Coastal Goods, Nantucket, Cape Cod, MA. Salt Sensations (seasoned sea salts): www.coastalgoods.com

▶ Espana Sea Salts, imported by Power Seller Imports, Seattle, WA: www.psimports.net

▶ The Spice Hut, Bellingham, WA. Indian spices, flavored sea salts and teas; order by phone or on their website: Phone 360-671-2800; www.thespicehut.com

AUTHOR'S WEBSITES

▶ Anne Mikkelsen. Provides current links to emerging food science, new antioxidant/anti-inflammatory recipes, garden news, more stories, and ways to "spice up your life": www.annecuttermikkelsen.com

▶ Carolyn Stinson, marketing communications strategist and implementer, public and media relations counselor, author, writer: www.stinsonmarketing.com

Index